Handbook of Lower Extremity Reconstruction

Scott T. Hollenbeck
Editor

Peter B. Arnold • Dennis P. Orgill
Associate Editors

Handbook of Lower Extremity Reconstruction

Clinical Case-Based Review and Flap Atlas

Springer

Editor
Scott T. Hollenbeck
Plastic and Reconstructive
Surgery
Duke Medical Center
Durham, NC
USA

Associate Editors
Peter B. Arnold
Plastic and Reconstructive
Surgery
University of Mississippi
Medical Center
Jackson, MS
USA

Dennis P. Orgill
Division of Plastic Surgery
Brigham and Women's Hospital
Harvard Medical School
Boston, MA
USA

ISBN 978-3-030-41034-6 ISBN 978-3-030-41035-3 (eBook)
https://doi.org/10.1007/978-3-030-41035-3

This Springer imprint is published by the registered company Springer Nature Switzerland AG
The registered company address is: Gewerbestrasse 11, 6330 Cham, Switzerland

To our families for their support and patience. To our teachers for their effort and knowledge. To our patients for their trust and resilience. To our trainees for always questioning and pushing forward. To our assistants and partners for having our back.

Scott T. Hollenbeck
Peter B. Arnold
Dennis P. Orgill

Preface

I often ask residents and students to define the goal of lower extremity reconstruction. I hear all kinds of answers from "limb salvage" to "return to work" to "bony healing." At the end of the day, I think the goal of lower extremity reconstruction can best be summarized simply as "painless ambulation." If this goal is achieved, then the reconstructive surgeon has done their patient a service.

In this book, you will find a broad range of topics designed to prepare surgeons who will encounter lower extremity wounds. As the majority of reconstructive lower extremity wounds are traumatic in nature, we focus primarily on trauma care. However, important topics such as diabetic limb salvage, nonsurgical wound care, and oncologic reconstruction are also covered. The book is divided into two parts. Section I consists of concepts and anatomic region-specific discussions. Section II is essentially an atlas for performing flaps for the lower extremity. Rather than simply showing how to dissect a given flap, the atlas is unique in that it is defect based. For example, a defect of the knee is shown, and several flap options are presented for that specific problem. In my mind, this is far more practical than a flap dissection guide.

The atlas's illustrations are meant to show the key steps in setting up and raising the flap for a given defect. We realize there are many ways to do each flap and to address each problem. What we have presented here is what we believe to be *the most practical and reliable approach*. Certainly, extreme options and sophisticated approaches exist. Many of those esoteric approaches are best for the surgeon who has achieved expert status.

We hope this book will be useful to those "on the front line" – residents seeing consults in the emergency room, students preparing for plastic surgery or orthopedics rotations, and attending surgeons embarking on a comprehensive reconstructive clinical practice. Whatever the circumstance may be, we designed this book to help readers deliver real-time care. With hard work and perseverance, achieving painless ambulation for your patients is an attainable and worthwhile goal.

Durham, NC, USA Scott T. Hollenbeck, MD
Jackson, MS, USA Peter B. Arnold, MD
Boston, MA, USA Dennis P. Orgill, MD, PhD

Acknowledgments

The authors would like to acknowledge the pioneering work of John B. McCraw and Phillip G. Arnold. Their flap atlas has inspired many and remains a useful resource and true work of art. This book would not exist without the dedication and tireless work of our esteemed colleagues who contributed valuable time and effort to writing chapters and generating figures. We have selected some of the most well-known lower extremity surgeons and teachers to contribute. Finally, we would like to acknowledge the tireless work of Lee Klein and his team at Springer for making this book a reality.

Contents

Part I Clinical

1 **Introduction to Lower Extremity Reconstruction: Historical Perspectives, Advances in the Field, and the Future** 3
Saïd C. Azoury and L. Scott Levin

2 **Essential Anatomy of the Lower Extremity** 13
Artur Fahradyan and Ketan M. Patel

3 **The Traumatized Leg** 43
Rachel E. Hein, Rose Tillis, and Howard Levinson

4 **Orthopaedic Principles of Lower Extremity Injuries** 55
Lily R. Mundy, Daniel J. Cunningham, and Mark J. Gage

5 **Reconstruction of Oncologic Defects** 67
Franca Kraenzlin and Justin M. Sacks

6 **Reconstruction of the Diabetic Limb** 79
Hyunsuk Peter Suh and Joon Pio (Jp) Hong

7 **Technological Advances to Simplify Lower Extremity Reconstruction** 93
Dennis P. Orgill and Mahendra Daya

8 Flap Principles Applied to Lower Extremity Reconstruction 101
Bryan J. Pyfer, Rebecca Vernon, and Scott T. Hollenbeck

9 Local Skin Flaps for Lower Extremity Wounds 115
Dennis P. Orgill, Andrew Atia, and Scott T. Hollenbeck

10 Principles of Local Muscle Flaps for Lower Extremity Wounds 129
Andrew L. Peredo, Matthew L. Iorio, and David W. Mathes

11 Soft Tissue Reconstruction of the Thigh 139
Trevor C. Hansen and Derek E. Bell

12 Knee and Proximal Lower Leg Wounds 149
Benjamin Googe, Somjade J. Songcharoen, and Peter B. Arnold

13 Soft Tissue Reconstruction of the Middle Third of the Leg 157
Katherine C. Benedict and Benjamin McIntyre

14 Soft Tissue Reconstruction of the Distal Third of the Lower Extremity 167
Roger W. Cason, Jonah P. Orr, and Suhail K. Mithani

15 Soft Tissue Reconstruction of the Foot 181
Whitney O. Lane, Ronnie L. Shammas, and Scott T. Hollenbeck

16 Amputation Principles and Targeted Muscle Reinnervation 195
Sean Figy, Ryan C. Jefferson, and Ian L. Valerio

Part II Flap Atlas

17 Soft Tissue Reconstruction of the Medial Thigh and Groin 215
Andrew L. Peredo, Victoria Wickenheisser, Caitlin Elizabeth Marks, and Scott T. Hollenbeck

18 Soft Tissue Reconstruction of the Lateral Thigh and Hip 237
Mahsa Taskindoust and Scott T. Hollenbeck

19 Soft Tissue Reconstruction of the Distal Thigh and Proximal Knee 245
Victoria Wickenheisser and Scott T. Hollenbeck

20 Soft Tissue Reconstruction for the Knee and Proximal Tibia 257
Victoria Wickenheisser, Benjamin Googe, and Scott T. Hollenbeck

21 Soft Tissue Reconstruction of the Middle Third of the Tibia 263
Benjamin Googe, Somjade J. Songcharoen, and Peter B. Arnold

22 Soft Tissue Reconstruction of the Distal Third Tibia 273
Benjamin Googe, Somjade J. Songcharoen, and Peter B. Arnold

23 Soft Tissue Reconstruction of the Foot 285
Benjamin Googe, Somjade J. Songcharoen, and Peter B. Arnold

24 Recipient Vessels for Lower Extremity Free Flap Reconstruction 295
Kate B. Krucoff and Scott T. Hollenbeck

Index 303

Contributors

Peter B. Arnold, MD, PhD, FACS Division of Plastic and Reconstructive Surgery, University of Mississippi Medical Center, Jackson, MS, USA

Andrew Atia, MD Division of Plastic and Reconstructive Surgery, Duke University Medical Center, Durham, NC, USA

Saïd C. Azoury, MD Division of Plastic Surgery, University of Pennsylvania, Philadelphia, PA, USA

Derek E. Bell, MD Division of Plastic and Reconstructive Surgery, University of Rochester Medical Center, Rochester, NY, USA

Katherine C. Benedict, MD Division of Plastic and Reconstructive Surgery, University of Mississippi Medical Center, Jackson, MS, USA

Roger W. Cason, MD Division of Plastic, Maxillofacial, and Oral Surgery, Duke University Health System, Durham, NC, USA

Daniel J. Cunningham, MD, MHSc Department of Orthopaedic Surgery, Duke University, Durham, NC, USA

Mahendra Daya, MD Department of Plastic and Reconstructive Surgery, Inkosi Albert Luthuli Central Hospital, Mayville, South Africa

Artur Fahradyan, MD Division of Plastic and Reconstructive Surgery, University of Southern California, Los Angeles, CA, USA

Sean Figy, MD Department of Surgery, The University of Nebraska Medical Center, Omaha, NE, USA

Mark J. Gage, MD Department of Orthopaedic Surgery, Duke University, Durham, NC, USA

Benjamin Googe, MD Division of Plastic and Reconstructive Surgery, University of Mississippi Medical Center, Jackson, MS, USA

Trevor C. Hansen, MD Division of Plastic and Reconstructive Surgery, University of Rochester Medical Center, Rochester, NY, USA

Rachel E. Hein, MD Department of Surgery, Division of Plastic Surgery, Duke University Medical Center, Durham, NC, USA

Scott T. Hollenbeck, MD, FACS Division of Plastic and Reconstructive Surgery, Duke Medical Center, Durham, NC, USA

Matthew L. Iorio, MD Division of Plastic Surgery, University of Colorado Hospital, Aurora, CO, USA

Ryan C. Jefferson, MD Department of Plastic and Reconstructive Surgery, The Ohio State University Wexner Medical Center, Columbus, OH, USA

Franca Kraenzlin, MD Department of Plastic Surgery, Johns Hopkins Hospital, Owings Mills, MD, USA

Kate B. Krucoff, MD Division of Plastic and Reconstructive Surgery, Duke University Medical Center, Durham, NC, USA

Whitney O. Lane, MD Division of Plastic, Maxillofacial, and Oral Surgery, Duke University Medical Center, Durham, NC, USA

L. Scott Levin, MD, FACS Department of Orthopaedic Surgery, Department of Surgery (Plastic Surgery), University of Pennsylvania, Philadelphia, PA, USA

Howard Levinson, MD, FACS Departments of Surgery, Pathology, and Dermatology, Duke University Medical Center, Durham, NC, USA

Caitlin Elizabeth Marks Duke University School of Medicine, Duke University, Durham, NC, USA

David W. Mathes, MD Department of Surgery, Division of Plastic and Reconstructive Surgery, University of Colorado, Anschutz Medical Campus, Aurora, CO, USA

Benjamin McIntyre, MD, FACS Division of Plastic and Reconstructive Surgery, University of Mississippi Medical Center, Jackson, MS, USA

Suhail K. Mithani, MD Division of Plastic, Maxillofacial, and Oral Surgery, Duke University Health System, Durham, NC, USA

Lily R. Mundy, MD Division of Plastic and Reconstructive Surgery, Duke University, Durham, NC, USA

Jonah P. Orr, BS Division of Plastic, Maxillofacial, and Oral Surgery, Duke University Health System, Durham, NC, USA

Dennis P. Orgill, MD, PhD, FACS Division of Plastic Surgery, Brigham & Women's Hospital, Harvard Medical School, Boston, MA, USA

Ketan M. Patel, MD Division of Plastic and Reconstructive Surgery, University of Southern California, Los Angeles, CA, USA

Andrew L. Peredo, MD Department of Surgery, Division of Plastic and Reconstructive Surgery, University of Colorado, Anschutz Medical Campus, Aurora, CO, USA

Joon Pio (Jp) Hong, MD, PhD, MBA Department of Plastic and Reconstructive Surgery, Asan Medical Center, University of Ulsan College of Medicine, Seoul, South Korea

Bryan J. Pyfer, MD, MBA Division of Plastic Surgery, Duke University Hospital, Durham, NC, USA

Justin M. Sacks, MD, MBA, FACS Department of Plastic and Reconstructive Surgery, Johns Hopkins School of Medicine, Baltimore, MD, USA

Ronnie L. Shammas, MD Division of Plastic, Maxillofacial, and Oral Surgery, Duke University Health System, Durham, NC, USA

Somjade J. Songcharoen, MD Division of Plastic and Reconstructive Surgery, University of Mississippi Medical Center, Jackson, MS, USA

Hyunsuk Peter Suh, MD Department of Plastic and Reconstructive Surgery, Asan Medical Center, University of Ulsan College of Medicine, Seoul, South Korea

Mahsa Taskindoust Levine Science Research Center, Duke University, Durham, NC, USA

Rose Tillis, MD Division of Plastic and Reconstructive Surgery, Duke University Hospital, Durham, NC, USA

Ian L. Valerio, MD, MS, MBA, FACS Division of Burn, Wound, and Trauma, Departments of Plastic and Reconstructive, General, and Orthopaedic Surgery, The Ohio State University Wexner Medical Center, Columbus, OH, USA

Rebecca Vernon, MD Division of Plastic, Maxillofacial, and Oral Surgery, Duke University School of Medicine, Durham, NC, USA

Victoria Wickenheisser, MD Division of Plastic and Reconstructive Surgery, Duke University Hospital, Durham, NC, USA

Part I
Clinical

Chapter 1
Introduction to Lower Extremity Reconstruction: Historical Perspectives, Advances in the Field, and the Future

Saïd C. Azoury and L. Scott Levin

Reconstruction of the lower extremity has evolved as a separate discipline within reconstructive surgery. Trauma is the most common etiology for lower extremity wounds that require reconstruction, followed by tumor resection, infection, or underlying vascular disease. Patients with peripheral vascular disease or diabetes often develop wounds that require débridement, skeletal stabilization, and soft tissue coverage. Regardless of the etiology, the goal of reconstruction is to restore form as well as function.

S. C. Azoury
Division of Plastic Surgery, University of Pennsylvania, Philadelphia, PA, USA

L. S. Levin (✉)
Department of Orthopaedic Surgery, Department of Surgery (Plastic Surgery), University of Pennsylvania, Philadelphia, PA, USA
e-mail: Lawrence.Levin2@uphs.upenn.edu

S. T. Hollenbeck et al. (eds.), *Handbook of Lower Extremity Reconstruction*, https://doi.org/10.1007/978-3-030-41035-3_1

Background

Understanding the concept of the reconstructive ladder as it relates to the lower extremity is critical (Fig. 1.1) [1, 2]. Non-flap closure (*eg*, complex closure, grafting) or rotational flaps represent the lower rungs on the ladder and are most useful for smaller defects. For larger defects, free-tissue transfer may be the best option; it represents one of the higher rungs on the reconstructive ladder. The most common recipient site for free flap reconstruction of the leg is the distal third of the extremity, including the ankle and foot, where options for local flaps are limited. Further adding to the complexity of the treatment algorithm, the characteristics of a wound may alter the usual reconstructive options for any given location. For instance, a defect on the proximal third of the leg that is typically addressed with a pedicled gastrocnemius muscle flap may require free flap coverage in the setting of large composite-type defects.

Lower extremity reconstruction requires multidisciplinary care. Orthopaedic and plastic surgeons must be supported by musculoskeletal radiologists, vascular surgeons, infectious disease specialists, physical therapists, prosthetists, and specialized nursing staff [3]. In addition to the surgical treatment of lower extremity wounds, the psychosocial component is equally important, as the success of these patients depends on a strong support system. Psychiatrists and pain management are integral to any lower extremity treatment team. The reconstructed extremity must be able to bear weight, but not at the expense of insufferable pain. The postoperative phase is often the longest part of the treatment, and physical and occupational rehabilitation are fundamental to a successful recovery.

Historical Perspectives

The treatment of lower extremity wounds has evolved since the teachings of Hippocrates during Greece's Classical period nearly 2500 years ago. Similar to modern practice, fractures

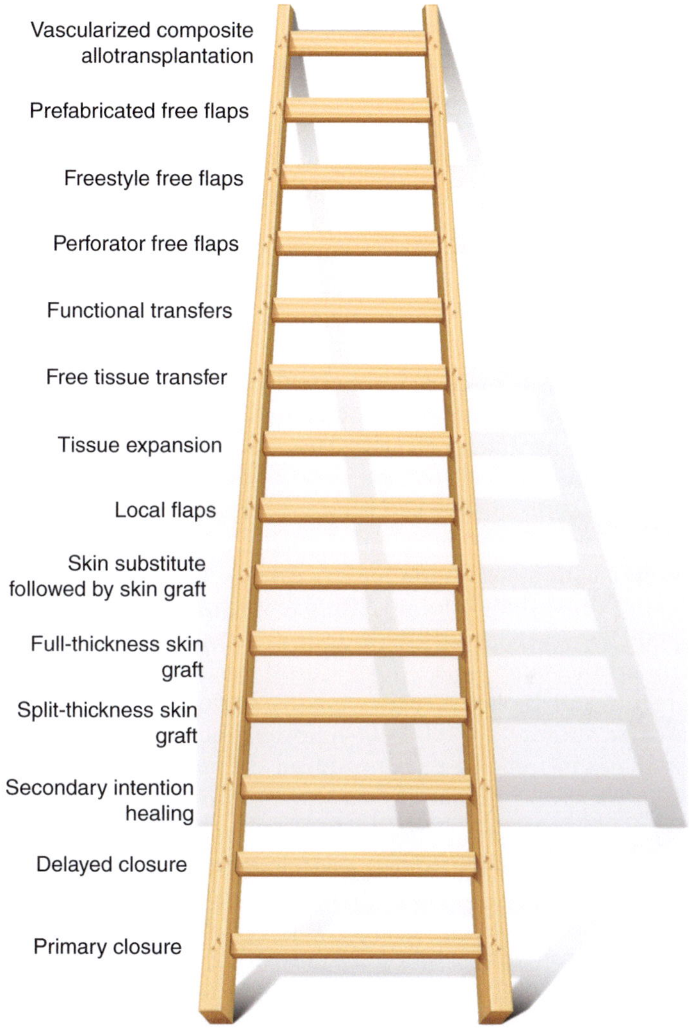

FIGURE 1.1 Reconstructive ladder for lower extremity soft tissue defects

were stabilized with splints or external fixators, but soft tissue wounds were treated with ointments and potions. Hippocrates also described therapeutic amputation for vascular gangrene, while leaving the wound open to heal by secondary intention. Nearly four centuries later, Celsus wrote about the cardinal signs of inflammation: rubor, calor, dolor, tumor. He emphasized the need for early débridement of a wound, removal of foreign bodies, and hemostasis. In the mid sixteenth century, Ambroise Paré, a French surgeon considered one of the fathers of surgery, described the continuing pain of an amputated limb, so-called phantom limb. Pain continues to be a driver of discussion when considering early amputation and prosthetic fitting or complex limb salvage.

Significant progress in the field of lower extremity reconstruction was made in the twentieth century. Thomas Huntington (1849–1929) was well known for his contributions to aseptic surgery as well as the treatment of fractures. In 1905, he was presented with a challenging case of a young boy left with a substantial defect following radical debridement of tibial shaft osteomyelitis. He was the first to perform a pedicled vascularized fibula graft to reconstruct the defect. Around the same time, Alexis Carrel (1873–1944), a French surgeon and biologist, was studying various techniques in vascular surgery. In 1902, he reported the first end-to-end vascular anastomosis and introduced the concept of triangulation for vessel repair. He was awarded the Nobel prize in 1912 for his work, which set the foundation for the burgeoning field of microvascular reconstruction in the latter half of the twentieth century. Sir Harold Gillies (1882–1960) is widely accepted as the father of modern plastic and reconstructive surgery. Through his experience in treating wounded soldiers in World War I, he developed many of the techniques for reconstructing damaged tissues. Many believe that the so-called orthoplastic discipline traces back to 1919, when the Introduction for Gillies' plastic surgery textbook was written by an orthopaedic surgeon, Sir W. Arbuthnot Lane. In 1946, W.J. Stark described the first pedicled muscle flap to treat lower extremity osteomyelitis. In his experience, Stark observed that the use of a pedicled muscle flap along with débridement and antibiotics had double the success rate for treating chronic osteomyelitis, compared with no flap.

Countless advancements were made in vascularized bone, soft tissue flaps, and microsurgical techniques in the latter half of the twentieth century. In the late 1950s, Dr. Harry Buncke (1922–2008) served as a Senior Registrar at the Plastic Surgical and Burn Unit in Glasgow, Scotland. There, he was deeply influenced by Thomas Gibson (1915–1993) in vascular reconstruction and transplantation. Upon returning to the United States, he began using his newly acquired knowledge and made possible the replantation and transfer of tissues fed by 1-mm vessels. Around the same time, Julius Jacobsen and his student, Ernesto Suarez, found themselves dissatisfied with the magnification offered by surgical loupes. They introduced the operating microscope for small vessel anastomosis in 1960. In 1972, McGregor and Jackson described a new axial flap, the groin flap, and 1973, Rollin Daniel and G. Ian Taylor reported the first free groin flap transfer to cover a lower extremity soft tissue defect. In 1975, G. Ian Taylor described the first use of a free vascularized fibula for large segmental bone defects, which added yet another tool for the reconstructive surgeon. In an article that they coauthored, Daniel and Taylor opened by referencing Harry Buncke: “The successful transplantation of a block of composite tissue by reanastomosing the microvascular pedicle has untold experimental and clinical possibilities” [4]. The clinical impact of these historical milestones would soon be appreciated in the years that followed.

Composite vascularized tissue transfers became commonplace in the 1980s, and Marko Godina (1943–1986) was yet another pioneer in the field of lower extremity reconstructive microsurgery [5, 6]. His ideas lead to the first temporary ectopic implantation of an amputated hand and subsequent replantation after wound stability (Fig. 1.2). He also reported the first clinical use of free lateral arm flap, microvascular latissimus dorsi muscle flap, and saphenous neurovascular flap. In 1986, the year of his passing, he described the pathophysiology of

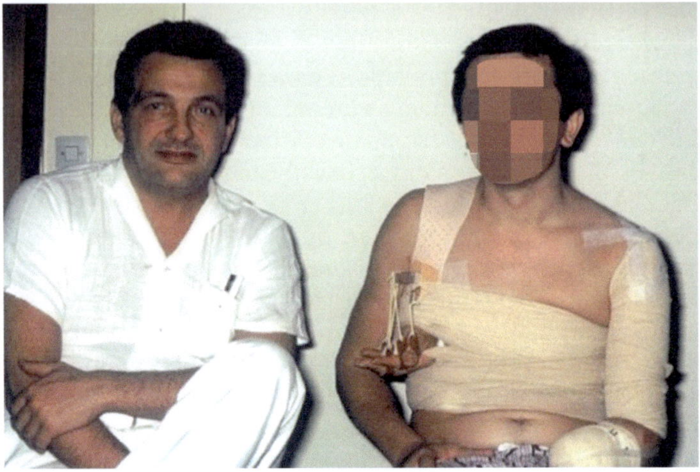

Figure 1.2 Dr. Marko Godina (*left*) was a pioneer in reconstructive microsurgery. His innovative ideas led to the first ectopic transplantation of a mutilated upper extremity for later replantation. (*Courtesy of* Photo Archive Medicina Danes)

high-energy trauma and advocated for radical débridement and early tissue coverage within the first 3 days after injury [7]. He also supported the practice of end-to-side anastomosis over end-to-end, in order to preserve distal blood flow in lower extremity microvascular reconstruction. These principles continue to guide our practice today.

Advances in the Field

Over the past several decades, the chronic complications of limb salvage surgery have been osteomyelitis and nonunion. The "Godina method" of treating complex lower extremity wounds with early radical débridement, skeletal fixation, and soft tissue coverage has stood the test of time in reducing these complications. Along with systemic antibiotics, the use of antibiotic-impregnated cement was introduced in order to administer antibiotics at higher concentrations locally than could be achieved via intravenous routes [5]. This method was used by orthopaedic surgeons in the 1970s and remains useful in lower extremity reconstruction.

Health care systems are becoming highly specialized in the coordinated care of patients requiring lower extremity reconstruction. The collaborative approach between orthopaedic and plastic surgeons for the past quarter of a century has evolved, resulting in a unique field of reconstructive surgery—orthoplastic surgery. Fellowships are now available to train not only aspiring microsurgeons, but also those individuals with a particular interest in orthoplastic surgery.

Advances in diagnostic imaging, such as CT angiography, MRI/MRA, and ultrasonography, have allowed for better detection of vascular compromise that should be addressed prior to reconstruction [8]. Many patients who require reconstruction for lower extremity wounds have underlying vascular disease. Impaired vascular flow also inhibits the healing of small defects secondary to trauma, surgical incisions, infection, or vascular ulcers, which may ultimately result in extensive defects that require free flap coverage. These imaging modalities also help to delineate the anatomy for choosing flap recipient vessels and provide information regarding superficial and deep venous outflow.

Negative pressure wound therapy (NPWT) was introduced in 1995 and has become widely embraced across various surgical specialties for acute and chronic wounds [9]. It has improved the management of lower extremity wounds and fracture care. NPWT can safely be placed on select composite defects and promotes formation of granulation tissue needed for skin grafting. NPWT functions to remove wound exudate, thereby optimizing conditions for wound healing. Although NPWT serves multiple purposes in the treatment of lower extremity wounds, it is never a substitute for vascularized tissue transfer. Dermal matrices were originally developed for burn reconstruction, but they are now used as an adjunct that can be employed to cover large areas of tissue with underlying exposed bone and tendon, which previously were not considered amenable for skin grafting. When applied to superficial wounds, the aesthetic results are comparable to other methods of reconstruction.

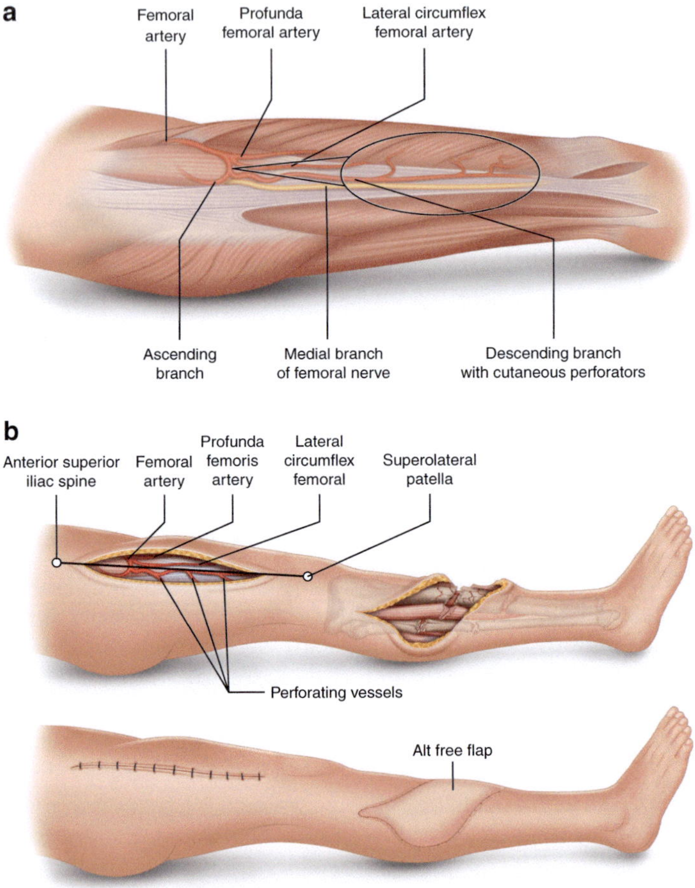

FIGURE 1.3 Use of perforator flap, specifically the fasciocutaneous anterolateral thigh (ALT) flap, for lower extremity trauma reconstruction. (**a**), The anterolateral thigh flap is based on the descending branch of the lateral femoral circumflex artery. The advantages of using ALT perforator flap (**b**) include reduced donor site morbidity, with an incision that can often be closed primarily, as well as a large skin paddle for coverage

The increased use of perforator flaps has revolutionized the reconstructive armamentarium (Fig. 1.3). Perforator flaps reduce donor site morbidity and have improved overall patient satisfaction following limb salvage. Greater attention is being paid to improving the aesthetics of reconstructive efforts, using techniques such as endoscopic tissue expansion to release contractures or remove skin grafts that were used to close fasciotomy wounds.

Future Directions

Even with the advances that have been made in lower extremity reconstruction, efforts may fail as a result of risks described nearly a century ago. Continuing to critically review limb salvage techniques will provide additional evidence to guide practice. Strengthening infrastructure for reconstruction has been shown to correlate with improved outcomes and decreased costs. Promoting the value of a multidisciplinary approach, specifically orthoplastic surgery, will result in a higher rate of successful limb salvage in patients at risk for amputation.

The success of prosthetics and composite tissue allotransplantation will have a significant impact on the long-term future of lower extremity reconstruction. Although we are making progress in upper extremity transplantation, lower extremity transplantation at this time does not justify the risks associated with long-term immunosuppression. When considering the most severe cases of trauma, outcomes following salvage are similar to those after amputation, and decision-making continues to be guided by patient preference and provider expertise. Scoring systems have been developed as a way to assist the surgical team in deciding on amputation versus salvage [10], but their clinical utility has not been validated. A future goal should be to better predict those who would perform better with reconstruction or amputation and prosthesis. Until amputation and myoelectric prosthesis prove to be functionally better, safer, and more cost-effective than limb salvage, reconstruction will continue to be a viable option preferred by many patients. For this reason, plastic and orthopaedic surgeons must continue to be trained in complex and microsurgical reconstruction in order to be prepared to deliver the best care possible to these patients. The following chapters provide a comprehensive guide to lower extremity reconstruction, with detailed descriptions of the various approaches used based on the wound characteristics and location.

References

1. Sbitany H, Au AF, Kovach SJ, Levin LS. Lower limb functional reconstruction. In: Pu LLQ, Levine JP, Wei F-C, editors. Reconstructive surgery of the lower extremity. St. Louis: Quality Medical Publishing; 2013. p. 1025–45.
2. Tintle SM, Levin LS. The reconstructive microsurgery ladder in orthopaedics. Injury. 2013;44:376–85.
3. Lerman OZ, Kovach SJ, Levin LS. The respective roles of plastic and orthopedic surgery in limb salvage. Plast Reconstr Surg. 2011;127:215S–27S.
4. Daniel RK, Taylor GI. Distant transfer of an island flap by microvascular anastomoses: a clinical technique. Plast Reconstr Surg. 1973;52:111–7.
5. Colen DL, Colen LB, Levin LS, Kovach SJ. Godina's principles in the twenty-first century and the evolution of lower extremity trauma reconstruction. J Reconstr Microsurg. 2018;34:563–71.
6. Hong JPJ, Colen LB. How has Dr. Marko Godina influenced us? Plast Reconstr Surg. 2017;140:641–2.
7. Godina M. Early microsurgical reconstruction of complex trauma of the extremities. Plast Reconstr Surg. 1986;78:285–92.
8. Fang F, Lin CH. Lower extremity reconstruction. In: Wei F-C, Mardini S, editors. Flaps and reconstructive surgery. 2nd ed. New York: Elsevier; 2017. p. 255–74.
9. Gerry R, Kwei S, Bayer L, Breuing KH. Silver-impregnated vacuum-assisted closure in the treatment of recalcitrant venous stasis ulcers. Ann Plast Surg. 2007;59:58–62.
10. Higgins TF, Klatt JB, Beals TC. Lower Extremity Assessment Project (LEAP)—the best available evidence on limb-threatening lower extremity trauma. Orthop Clin North Am. 2010;41:233–9.

Chapter 2
Essential Anatomy of the Lower Extremity

Artur Fahradyan and Ketan M. Patel

The lower extremity is often involved in trauma or other disease processes requiring reconstructive procedures in an attempt to maintain its anatomic and functional integrity. It also serves as a donor site for free flaps to reconstruct other body parts. Therefore, understanding the complex anatomy of the lower extremity is fundamental for every reconstructive surgeon to learn and understand. The aim of this chapter is to review the essentials of skeletal, muscular, fascial, and important neurovascular anatomic structures of the thigh, leg, and foot.

The Thigh

The thigh is an important tissue donor for commonly used local, regional, and free flaps, such as the gracilis and sartorius muscle flaps, and various perforator flaps. Therefore, knowing the thigh anatomy helps us to harvest these flaps for many reconstructive procedures.

A. Fahradyan · K. M. Patel (✉)
Division of Plastic and Reconstructive Surgery, University of Southern California, Los Angeles, CA, USA

S. T. Hollenbeck et al. (eds.), *Handbook of Lower Extremity Reconstruction*, https://doi.org/10.1007/978-3-030-41035-3_2

Thigh Skeletal Structure

The borders of the thigh extend from the infragluteal crease and the inguinal ligament to the tibiofemoral joint. The skeletal structure of the thigh is made up of a single femoral bone, which articulates with the pelvic acetabulum proximally in the hip joint, and with the tibia and the patella distally to make up the knee joint [1–4]. The femur receives direct endosteal and periosteal blood supply from multiple sources, but the most clinically relevant in terms of tissue reconstruction is the genicular arterial system to the distal metaphyseal region. Periosteum, cortical, and cancellous bone can be harvested from the medial femur as a vascularized flap using the descending genicular artery [2]. It is utilized as a free flap in treatment of bony nonunions of the clavicle, humerus, tibia, and radius.

Thigh Fascial Layers

The thigh has a superficial fascia and deep fascia. The superficial fascia lies within the subcutaneous fat, and the deep fascia lies below it. The deep fascia, also called the *investing fascia of the thigh* or *fascia lata*, encircles the thigh muscles. The superficial and deep fascial layers join at the inguinal ligament. The great saphenous vein, superficial branches of the femoral artery, and the lymphatic vessels transition from deep to superficial in this region, passing through the fossa ovalis, which is an opening in both fascial layers. The iliotibial tract, a thickening of the lateral aspect of the deep fascia that is attached to the tensor fascia latae muscle proximally, aids in maintaining knee extension [1–4].

Septa pass from the deep fascia to the femur, confining the thigh musculature within three compartments: anterior, posterior, and medial or adductor. It should be noted, however, that only the anterior and posterior compartments have fascial boundaries, whereas the adductor compartment is not a true anatomic compartment.

Thigh Musculature

The anterior (extensor) thigh compartment contains the following muscles:

- sartorius
- quadriceps femoris, which is composed of the rectus femoris, vastus lateralis, vastus intermedius and vastus medialis muscles (Table 2.1, Fig. 2.1).

The anterior compartment muscles extend the lower leg at the knee joint. In addition, the sartorius and rectus femoris muscles flex the thigh at the hip joint.

The sartorius muscle is a source for a commonly used local muscle and is often transposed to cover the proximal thigh wound with femoral vessel exposure. It is the most superficial muscle of the thigh and obliquely crosses the thigh from superolateral to inferomedial. The muscle originates from the anterior superior iliac spine and inserts on the proximal medial surface of the tibia. This is also an insertion point for the gracilis and semitendinosus muscles forming the pes anserinus [3, 4].

The quadriceps muscle originates from the femoral shaft. Its distal end makes up the quadriceps tendon, which crosses over the patella to become the patellar tendon and inserts onto the tibial tuberosity. One portion of the muscle can be removed to be used as a tissue donor. This is usually well tolerated with centralization of the remaining muscles and appropriate physical therapy. A portion of the vastus lateralis muscle is often taken with the anterolateral thigh flap, or the rectus femoris is used as a local flap with minimal or no functional deficit of the knee [5].

The posterior (flexor) thigh compartment contains these muscles:

- semitendinosus
- semimembranosus
- biceps femoris

TABLE 2.1 Overview of thigh musculature

	Muscle	Origin	Insertion	Function	Blood Supply	Innervation
Anterior compartment	Sartorius	Anterior superior iliac spine	Proximal medial tibia	Knee flexion and internal rotation Hip flexion, abduction and external rotation	SFA	Femoral
	Rectus femoris	Anterior superior iliac spine and ileum	Quadriceps tendon	Knee extension Hip flexion	LCFA SFA	Femoral
	Vastus lateralis	Femoral shaft	Quadriceps tendon	Knee extension	LCFA Direct branch from profunda femoris Superior genicular artery	Femoral
	Vastus medialis	Femoral shaft	Quadriceps tendon	Knee extension Patellar stabilization	SFA Descending genicular artery	Femoral
	Vastus intermedius	Femoral shaft	Quadriceps tendon	Knee extension	Direct branches from profunda femoris	Femoral

Posterior compartment	Biceps femoris	Long head-ischial tuberosity Short head-femur	Lateral tibial condyle and fibular head	Knee flexion and lateral rotation	Perforating branches of profunda femoris	Sciatic
	Semitendinosus	Ischial tuberosity	Proximal medial tibia	Hip extension Knee flexion and medial rotation	Perforating branches of profunda femoris SFA	Sciatic
	Semimembranosus	Ischial tuberosity	Medial tibial condyle	Hip extension Knee flexion and medial rotation	Perforating branches of profunda femoris Inferior gluteal artery MCFA Inferior medial genicular artery	Sciatic

(continued)

TABLE 2.1 (continued)

	Muscle	Origin	Insertion	Function	Blood Supply	Innervation
Medial compartment	Adductor magnus	Pubic bone	Femur	Hip adduction and internal rotation	Profunda femoris SFA	Obturator
	Adductor longus	Pubic bone	Femur	Hip adduction and internal rotation	Profunda femoris MCFA SFA	Obturator
	Adductor brevis	Pubic bone	Femur	Hip adduction	MCFA	Obturator
	Gracilis	Pubic bone	Proximal medial tibia	Hip adduction Knee flexion and internal rotation	MCFA SFA	Obturator
	Pectineus	Pubic bone	Femur	Hip adduction Knee flexion and internal rotation	MCFA	Femoral

LCFA lateral circumflex femoral artery, *MCFA* medial circumflex femoral artery, *SFA* superficial femoral artery

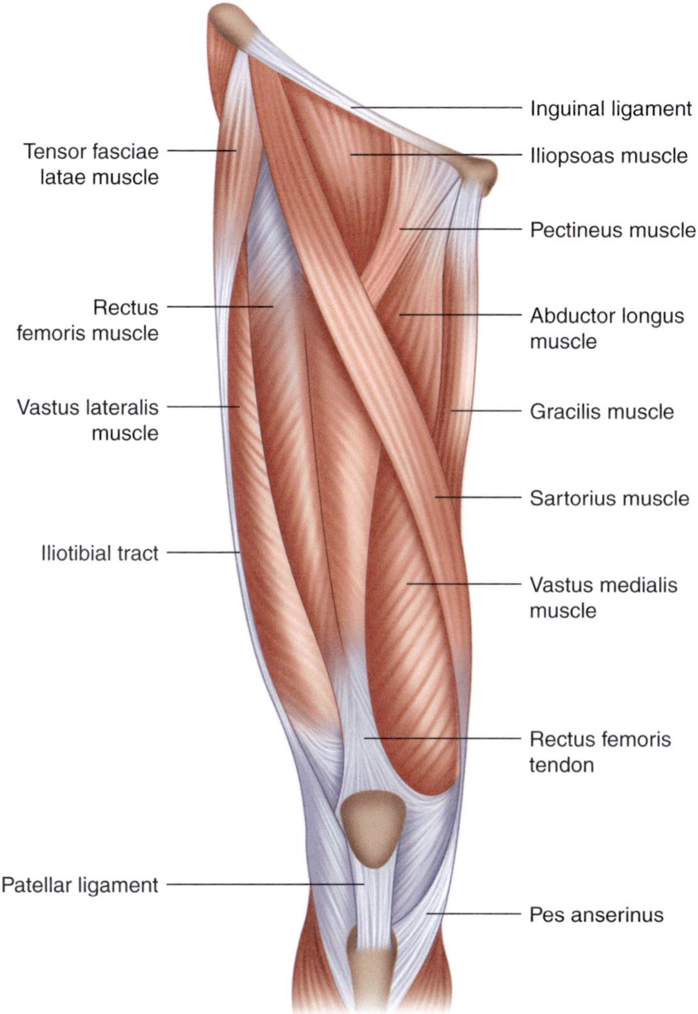

FIGURE 2.1 Muscles of thigh: anterior view

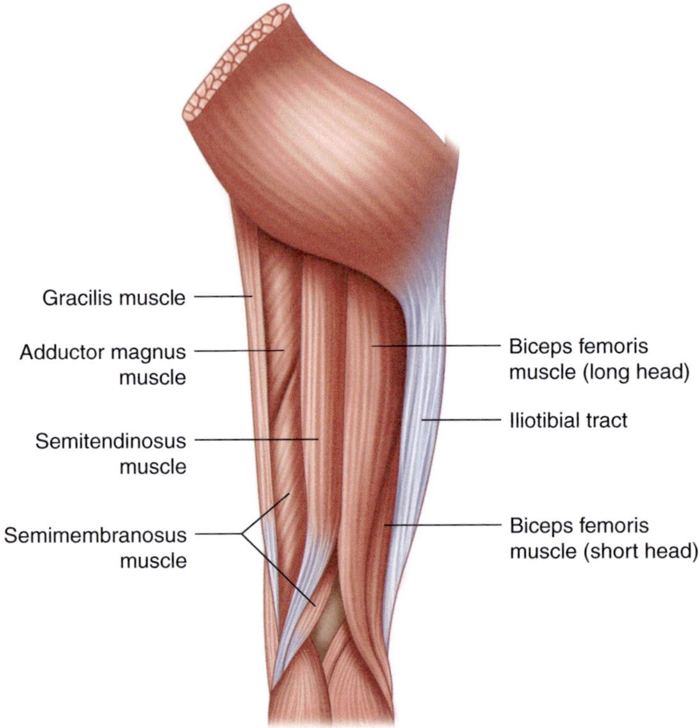

FIGURE 2.2 Muscles of thigh: posterior view

These are collectively known as the *hamstrings* and are knee flexors (Table 2.1, Fig. 2.2) [1–4]. The biceps femoris has two heads, the short and the long. The tendons of the semitendinosus and semimembranosus travel medially to form the superior medial border of the popliteal fossa, whereas the biceps femoris tendon travels laterally to form the superior lateral border of the popliteal fossa.

The medial (adductor) compartment contains these muscles:

- gracilis
- adductor magnus
- adductor brevis

- adductor longus
- pectineus

The gracilis muscle is commonly used as a free tissue donor site in reconstructive surgery. It is the most superficial muscle of the adductor compartment. It originates from the pubic bone and inserts into pes anserinus [6].

The tensor fascia latae is not classically included in any of the compartments of the thigh. It lies on the proximal lateral aspect of the thigh, originating from iliac crest, and usually ends at the proximal third of the lateral thigh.

Thigh Vascular System

The main blood supply to the lower extremity is via the femoral artery, which is the continuation of the external iliac artery below the inguinal ligament (Fig. 2.3). The femoral artery divides into two main branches approximately 4 cm below the inguinal canal:

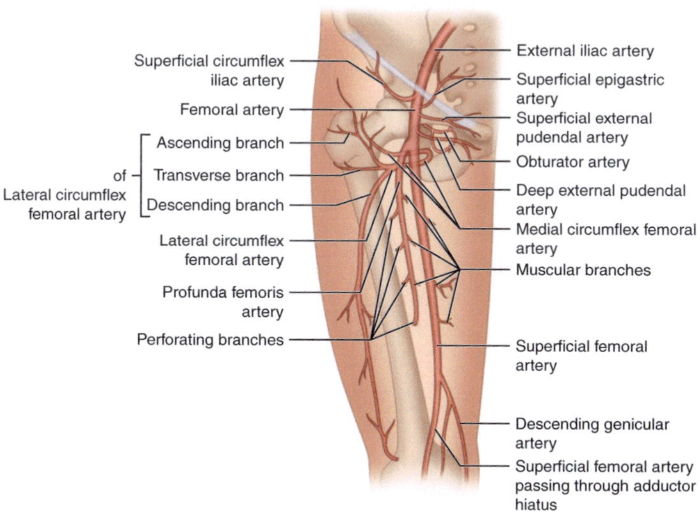

FIGURE 2.3 Major arteries of thigh

- superficial femoral artery
- profunda femoris artery

The superficial femoral artery provides blood supply to the thigh adductors, sartorius, and vastus medialis muscles as it passes beneath the sartorius muscle, travels in the Hunter's canal, exits through the adductor hiatus, and enters the popliteal fossa, where it becomes the popliteal artery.

The profunda femoris supplies the majority of the musculature of the thigh region. It has six main branches:

- medial circumflex femoral artery (transverse and descending branches)
- lateral circumflex femoral artery (ascending, transverse, and descending branches)
- four or more perforating branches

The medial circumflex femoral artery is usually the first major branch of the profunda femoris and supplies the adductor compartment. The transverse branch anastomoses with the transverse branch of the lateral circumflex femoral artery and the inferior gluteal artery posterior to the proximal femur. The descending branch splits into multiple muscular branches to supply the gracilis muscle.

The lateral circumflex arterial system, the second major branch of the profunda femoris artery, is important for reconstructive surgeons, as it provides several options for tissue harvesting. The ascending branch supplies the greater trochanter, the tensor fascia latae, the anterior iliac crest, and the skin overlying the hip region. The transverse branch passes through the vastus lateralis and anastomoses with the medial circumflex femoral artery posterior to the femoral head. The descending branch usually travels between the vastus intermedius and rectus femoris, giving septocutaneous or musculocutaneous perforating branches to the overlying skin. It should be noted that great variability of the lateral circumflex arterial system exists. Its takeoff can be in different locations on the profunda femoris in 20% of people. Occasionally it arises from the femoral artery itself (16%), presents as a split artery traveling from the femoral artery and the profunda femoris separately (3%), from the common origin for the profunda femoris and the medial circumflex femoral artery (5%), from the medial circumflex femoral artery (5%), or from other sites (4%). The anatomy of the cutaneous perforators also varies. Despite the anatomic variabilities of the lateral circumflex femoral arterial system, the proper dissection allows harvesting of multiple tissue flaps, such as anterolateral thigh, rectus femoris or tensor fascia latae muscle, iliac crest bone, or composite flaps.

The first perforating branch of the profunda femoris supplies the adductor brevis, adductor magnus, biceps femoris, and gluteus maximus muscles. The second, third, and fourth perforating branches supply the posterior compartment muscles.

Thigh Innervation

Three motor nerves supply the thigh musculature:

- femoral
- sciatic
- obturator

The femoral nerve provides motor innervation to the anterior compartment muscles. It arises from the L2–L4 nerve roots and divides into anterior and posterior divisions below the inguinal ligament. The anterior division provides motor innervation to the sartorius muscle, and the posterior division to the quadriceps femoris. The obturator nerve provides motor innervation to the medial compartment muscles. It arises from the L2–L4 spinal roots, enters the thigh via the obturator foramen, and splits into anterior and posterior branches. The anterior branch supplies the adductor longus, brevis, and gracilis muscles, and the posterior branch supplies the adductor magnus muscle. The sciatic nerve arises from the L4–S3 nerve roots, enters the posterior thigh via the sciatic foramen, and provides motor innervation to the posterior compartment musculature.

The cutaneous innervation to the thigh region comes from two pure sensory cutaneous nerves and the cutaneous branches from the femoral and obturator nerves:

- lateral femoral cutaneous nerve (pure sensory, arises from the lumbosacral plexus)
- posterior femoral cutaneous nerve (pure sensory, arises from the lumbosacral plexus)
- medial and intermediate cutaneous nerves (arise from the anterior division of the femoral nerve and innervate the medial thigh skin)
- sensory branches of the obturator nerve (innervate the inferomedial thigh)

The Leg

The leg extends from the knee to the ankle joints. The main function is the movement of the ankle and foot.

Leg Skeletal Structure

The leg skeletal structure is comprised of the medially placed tibia and lateral fibula. The tibia is the weight bearing bone in the leg, whereas the fibula mainly functions as muscle attachment sites and makes up the part of the ankle joint. The two bones are joined by a fibrous interosseous membrane. The tibia receives major endosteal blood supply through the proximal nutrient foramen near the soleus line. The periosteal blood supply to the tibial shaft arises from multiple segmental branches directly from anterior tibial artery and from perforators from the surrounding musculature. The fibula receives endosteal blood supply from a branch of the peroneal artery entering the bone via the nutrient foreman in the middle one-third of the shaft. It also receives a periosteal blood supply from multiple branches of the peroneal artery [1–4].

Leg Fascial Layers

The superficial fascia lies within the subcutaneous tissue. The great and lesser saphenous veins, as well as the sural and saphenous nerves travel along this layer. The deep fascia is the continuation of the fascia lata of the thigh and encircles the leg musculature. Intermuscular septa extending from the deep fascia divide the leg musculature into four compartments; anterior, lateral, superficial and deep posterior compartments which organize the leg musculature into similar functioning groups.

Leg Musculature

The anterior or the extensor compartment of the leg is comprised of 4 muscles (Table 2.2, Fig. 2.4)

- tibialis anterior
- extensor digitorum longus
- extensor hallucis longus
- peroneus tertius muscles

They are all responsible for ankle, foot and toe dorsiflexion. The tibialis anterior muscle originates from the lateral tibial condyle, the proximal two-thirds of the tibial shaft and the interosseous membrane and inserts on the inferomedial surface of the medial cuneiform and the base of the first metatarsal bone. Its function is foot dorsiflexion and inversion. The extensor digitorum longus has the same origin as the tibialis anterior and lies lateral to it. Its distal tendon divides into four slips that proceed to the second to fifth toes. It extends the toes, dorsiflexes synergistically with the tibialis anterior and extensor hallucis, as well as everts the foot. The extensor hallucis longus has the same origin but inserts on the base of the distal phalanx of the first toe. It dorsiflexes the first toe and foot. The peroneus tertius originates on the distal third of the fibula and inserts on the base of the fifth metatarsal bone.

Table 2.2 Overview of leg musculature

	Muscle	Origin	Insertion	Function	Blood Supply	Innervation
Anterior compartment	Tibialis anterior	Tibia and interosseous membrane	Medial cuneiform and interosseous membrane	Foot dorsiflexion and inversion	Anterior tibial	Deep peroneal
	Extensor digitorum longus	Fibula and interosseous membrane	Lateral four toes	Foot and 2nd–5th toe dorsiflexion and foot eversion	Anterior tibial	Deep peroneal
	Extensor hallucis longus	Fibula and interosseous membrane	Base of distal phalanx of big toe	1st toe dorsiflexion	Anterior tibial	Deep peroneal
	Peroneus tertius	Fibula and interosseous membrane	Base of 5th metatarsal	Foot dorsiflexion and eversion	Anterior tibial	Deep peroneal

Lateral compartment	Peroneus longus	Fibula	Base of 1st metatarsal and medial cuneiform	Foot plantarflexion and eversion	Peroneal	Superficial peroneal
	Peroneus brevis	Fibula	Base of 5th metatarsal	Foot plantarflexion and eversion	Peroneal	Superficial peroneal
Superficial posterior compartment	Medial gastrocnemius	Medial femoral condyle	Achilles tendon	Foot plantarflexion, leg flexion	Medial sural	Tibial
	Lateral gastrocnemius	Lateral femoral condyle	Achilles tendon	Foot plantarflexion, leg flexion	Lateral sural	Tibial
	Plantaris	Lateral supracondylar ridge of femur	Achilles tendon	Foot plantarflexion, leg flexion	Posterior tibial	Tibial
	Soleus	Shaft of tibia and fibula	Achilles tendon	Foot plantarflexion	Posterior tibial	Tibial

(continued)

Table 2.2 (continued)

	Muscle	Origin	Insertion	Function	Blood Supply	Innervation
Deep posterior compartment	Popliteus	Lateral condyle of femur	Medial tibia	Leg flexion, lateral rotation of femur on tibia	Medial and lateral genicular arteries	Tibial
	Flexor digitorum longus	Tibia	Distal phalanges of 2nd–5th toes	2nd–5th toe distal phalangeal flexion, foot plantarflexion	Posterior tibial	Tibial
	Flexor hallucis longus	Fibula	Base of distal phalanx of 1st toe	1st toe distal phalangeal flexion, foot plantarflexion	Posterior tibial	Tibial
	Tibialis posterior	Tibia and fibula, interosseous membrane	Tuberosity of navicular and medial cuneiform bones	Foot plantarflexion and inversion	Posterior tibial and peroneal	Tibial

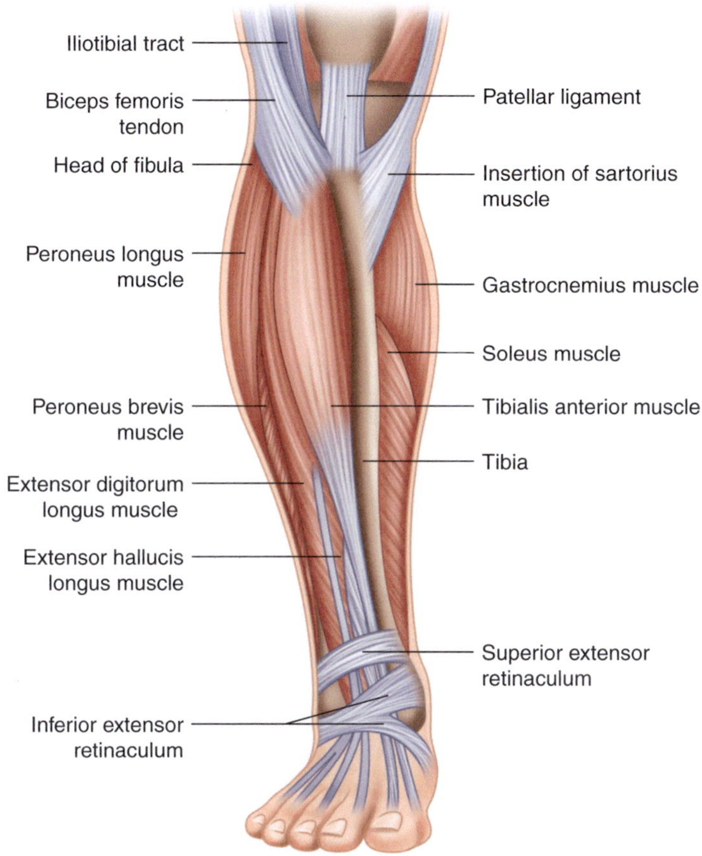

FIGURE 2.4 Leg muscles: anterior view

The lateral compartment is comprised of the (Table 2.2, Fig. 2.5)

- peroneus longus
- and brevis muscles.

They both originate from fibula. They convert into tendons at the ankle which travel behind the lateral malleolus. The peroneus brevis inserts on the base of the fifth metatarsal,

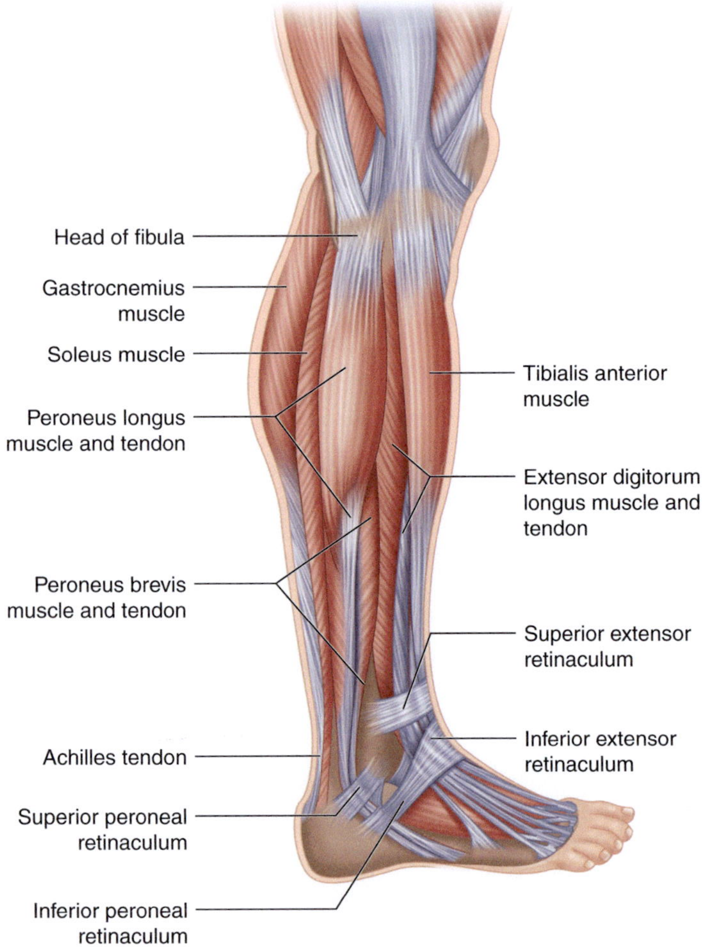

FIGURE 2.5 Leg muscles: lateral view

whereas the peroneus longus crosses the foot and inserts on the base of the first metatarsal bone. They are responsible for eversion and plantarflexion of the foot.

The posterior superficial compartment contains the (Table 2.2)

- medial and lateral gastrocnemius
- soleus
- and plantaris muscles.

The gastrocnemius and plantaris muscles originate on the femur and inserts on the calcaneus. They cause knee flexion and ankle plantarflexion. The proximal aspect of the medial and lateral gastrocnemius muscle heads forms the inferior border of the popliteal fossa. The gastrocnemius muscle is an important source of a local muscle flap for proximal leg soft tissue reconstruction [7]. The medial head is larger and longer than the lateral head and can cover larger defects. The plantaris muscle is a small muscle that lies between the gastrocnemius and soleus muscles. It has minimal functional activity and can be used as a source for tendon grafting. The soleus muscle works synergistically with the posterior compartment muscles to cause plantarflexion of foot. It originates from the proximal one-third of the tibia and posterior aspect of the fibular head. The tendons of the gastrocnemius, soleus and plantaris muscles coalesce to create the Achilles tendon which inserts into the posterior calcaneus. The superficial compartment muscles also act as muscle pumps to help with venous return.

The deep posterior compartment (deep flexor) contains (Table 2.2)

- the popliteus
- flexor digitorum longus
- flexor hallucis longus
- and tibialis posterior muscles.

They lie below the deep transverse fascia and cause knee flexion, toe flexion and foot plantarflexion upon activation. The popliteus muscle originates on the on the posterior aspect of the lateral femoral condyle and runs obliquely across the popliteal fossa to the posterior aspect of the proximal tibial shaft. It rotates the tibia medially on the femur to initiate knee flexion. The flexor digitorum longus originates from the tibia in the middle one-third of the leg extends down the leg behind the medial malleolus, crosses the sole of the foot and inserts on the plantar surfaces of the base of the distal phalanges. The flexor hallucis longus originates from the fibula in the middle one-third of the leg, travels down to the ankle and inserts onto the plantar surface of the distal phalanx of the first toe. The tibialis posterior muscle is the deepest muscle of the posterior deep complement. It originates from the proximal and mid one-third of the interosseous membrane and the surrounding tibia and fibula, courses down the leg, crosses the plantar surface of the foot and inserts into navicular and cuneiform bones.

Leg Vascular System

The vascular system of the leg derives from the popliteal artery, which is the continuation of the superficial femoral artery as it exits the Hunter's canal and enters the popliteal fossa. It gives off several important branches that supply the entire leg:

- large lateral branch
- superior medial and lateral genicular arteries
- middle genicular artery – supplies the posterior cruciate ligament
- medial and lateral sural arteries to the medial and lateral heads of the gastrocnemius muscle
- inferior medial and lateral genicular arteries
- anterior tibial artery
- peroneal artery
- posterior tibial artery

The superior lateral genicular artery connects with the descending branch of the lateral circumflex femoral artery, whereas the superior medial genicular artery with a branch directly from off the superficial femoral artery. The middle genicular artery supplies the posterior cruciate ligament.

The tibial artery is the first terminal branch of the popliteal artery as it exits the popliteal fossa. It passes through the superior aspect of the interosseous membrane to enter the anterior compartment and supplies all the muscles in this compartment. It then descends along the interosseous membrane, passes the ankle midway between the medial and lateral malleoli and becomes the dorsalis pedis artery.

The peroneal and posterior tibial arteries remain in the deep posterior compartment with peroneal artery running deeper and laterally closer to the fibula. The peroneal artery supplies the muscles in the lateral compartment. The posterior tibial artery descends down between the soleus and flexor digitorum longus muscles, becomes more superficial inferiorly and passes behind the medial malleolus to divide to its' terminal branches of medial and lateral plantar arteries. The posterior tibialis supplies all the muscles in the superficial and deep posterior compartments.

The vascular anatomy of the lower leg below the popliteal artery has some variations that is important to consider when planning lower extremity reconstructive procedures or harvesting free fibula flap based on peroneal artery to reconstruct defects in other anatomic locations. Kim-Lippert's classification is currently used in microvascular surgery to describe these anatomic variations [8]. In Type I and Type II variants the popliteal artery divides into its terminal branches proximal to the lower border of popliteus muscle (normal) and above the knee joint (high division) respectively, however, all three branches are fully developed. In Type III variant hypoplastic or aplastic branching with altered distal blood supply is present, which is further divided into 3 subtypes (Fig. 2.6)

- Type III – hypoplastic or aplastic branching
- IIIA – hypoplastic/aplastic posterior tibial artery
- IIIB – hypoplastic/aplastic anterior tibial artery
- IIIC – hypoplastic/aplastic anterior and posterior tibial arteries or peronea arteria magna

In Type III variant the peroneal artery plays a dominant role in providing blood supply to the leg and foot, therefore it is named dominant peroneal artery. This variation is present in 10% of population and 5.2% of any given limb. In 20% of people with dominant peroneal artery it is present in bilateral legs.

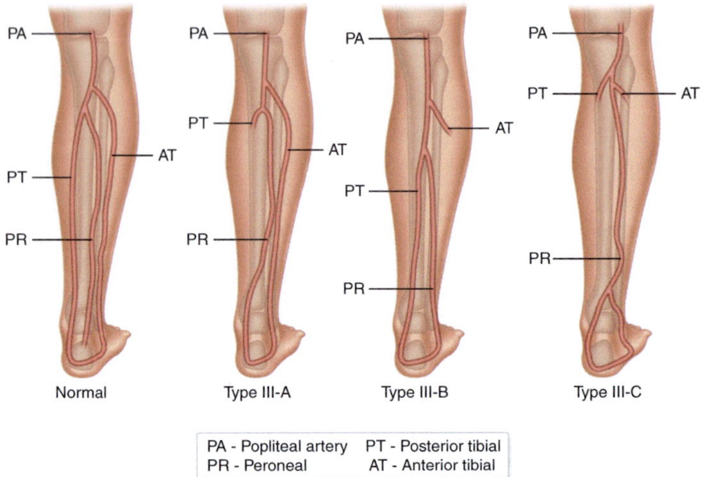

Figure 2.6 Leg vascular system: normal and type III variants

Leg Innervation

The sciatic nerve divides into

- tibial and
- common peroneal nerves

usually at the apex of the popliteal fossa and innervate the entire leg.

The tibial nerve descends down in the deep posterior compartment with posterior tibial artery and provides motor innervation to the musculature of superficial and deep posterior compartments. The medial and lateral motor sural nerves usually branch off in the distal portion of the proximal one-third of the popliteal fossa and reach the medial and lateral heads of the gastrocnemius muscle with medial and lateral sural arteries.

The common peroneal nerve curves lateral to the fibular neck and divides into two branches:

- superficial peroneal nerve
- deep peroneal nerve

The superficial peroneal nerve travels in the lateral leg compartment and provides motor innervation to the lateral compartment musculature. In the distal leg it becomes superficial and divides into medial and lateral branches which provide sensory innervation to the skin of the lower leg and foot. The deep peroneal nerve crosses medially from the lateral compartment to the anterior leg compartment and travels down along the interosseous membrane, behind the extensor digitorum longus. It innervates the muscles of the anterior compartment and the skin of the first dorsal webspace.

The skin of the leg is innervated by the sensory branches of the sciatic and femoral nerves and the posterior cutaneous nerve of the thigh:

- saphenous nerve – a branch of the femoral nerve, innervates the medial leg
- posterior femoral cutaneous nerve – branches directly from the sacral plexus, innervates posterior knee
- cutaneous branches of the superficial peroneal nerve – middle one-third of lateral leg and anterior ankle
- cutaneous branch of the deep peroneal nerve – first webspace, medial side of the second toe and lateral side of the great toe
- sural nerve – formed by the coalescing branches of the tibial (medial sural nerve) and common peroneal nerves (lateral sural nerve). It travels down the leg with lesser saphenous vein and innervates the distal on-third of the lateral leg skin. The medial and lateral sural nerves innervate the medial posterior and lateral postriot leg skin before they join to become the sural nerve. The sural nerve is easily located posterior to the lateral malleolus and is a common nerve harvest as a nerve graft.

The Ankle and Foot

The ankle and foot are highly functional parts of the lower extremity that require a detailed understanding of anatomy and function for proper reconstruction.

Ankle and Foot Skeletal Structure

The ankle comprises two joints [1]:

- articulation between the distal surfaces of fibula (lateral malleolus) and tibia (medial malleolus) with the superior aspect of the talus
- the subtalar joint – articulation between the inferior aspect of the talus with the calcaneus

The foot is comprised of

- tarsal bones
  - proximal row – the talus and calcaneus
  - distal row – the medial, intermediate and lateral cuneiform and the cuboid bones
  - navicular bone – between the talus and the cuneiform
- metatarsal bones
- toes
  - 1st toe – proximal and distal phalanges
  - 2nd – 5th toes – proximal, middle and distal phalanges

Ankle and Foot Fascial Layers

There are 3 major fascial retinacula in the ankle and foot (Figs. 2.4 and 2.5)

- the superior and inferior extensor retinacula – dorsum of foot, restricts the tibialis anterior, extensor hallucis longus, extensor digitorum longus and peroneus tertius tendons, the anterior tibial vessels and the deep peroneal nerve
- the flexor retinaculum – medial ankle, restrains the tibialis posterior, flexor digitorum longus and flexor hallucis longus tendons, the posterior tibial vessels and the tibial nerve
- the peroneal retinaculum – lateral ankle, retrains the peroneus longus and peroneus brevis tendons

The plantar fascia is a thick fibrous band attached to the calcaneus, divides into 5 bands distally which insert to the dermis beyond the metatarsal heads via retinacula cutis skin ligaments.

There are five major fascial compartments in the foot:

- four plantar compartments
  - medial – abductor hallucis and flexor hallucis brevis muscles
  - central – flexor digitorum brevis, lumbricals, flexor accessories and adductor hallucis muscles
  - lateral – abductor digiti minimi and flexor digiti minimi muscles
  - interosseous – seven interossei muscles
- one dorsal

Foot Musculature

There are intrinsic and extrinsic musculature that act on the foot and ankle [1–4]. The extrinsic muscles originate proximal to the foot, whereas all intrinsic muscles originate and insert within the foot and act mainly on toes.

The plantar muscles are organized in four layers (Figs. 2.7, 2.8, and 2.9)

- 1st layer is located beneath the plantar fascia and contains the flexor digitorum brevis, abductor hallucis and abductor digiti minimi muscles. They are all used in reconstructive surgery as local pedicled muscle flaps [9]
- 2nd layer is separated from the 1st layer by the tendons of flexor digitorum longus and flexor hallucis longus and contains flexor digitorum accessories (quadratus plantae muscle) and lumbricals [10]
- 3rd layer consists of the flexor hallucis brevis, adductor hallucis and flexor digiti minimi brevis muscles
- 4th layer contains three plantar interossei that adduct the toes and four dorsal interossei that abduct the toes

There are two dorsal muscles

- Extensor digitorum brevis used in reconstructive surgery as a local muscle flap for small foot and ankle defect based on lateral tarsal artery which is branch of dorsalis pedis.

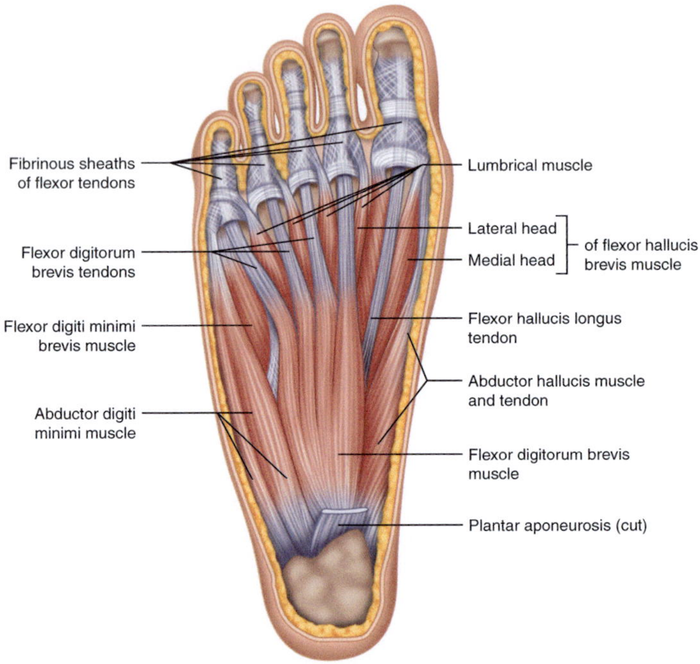

FIGURE 2.7 Muscles of sole of foot: first layer

- Extensor hallucis brevis

The loss of the dorsal muscle does not affect the function of the toes as the extension of the toes are mainly maintained by the extrinsic extensors.

Foot and Ankle Vascular System

There are three main vascular systems that supply the foot and ankle

- dorsalis pedis artery
- medial and lateral plantar arteries
- terminal branches of peroneal artery

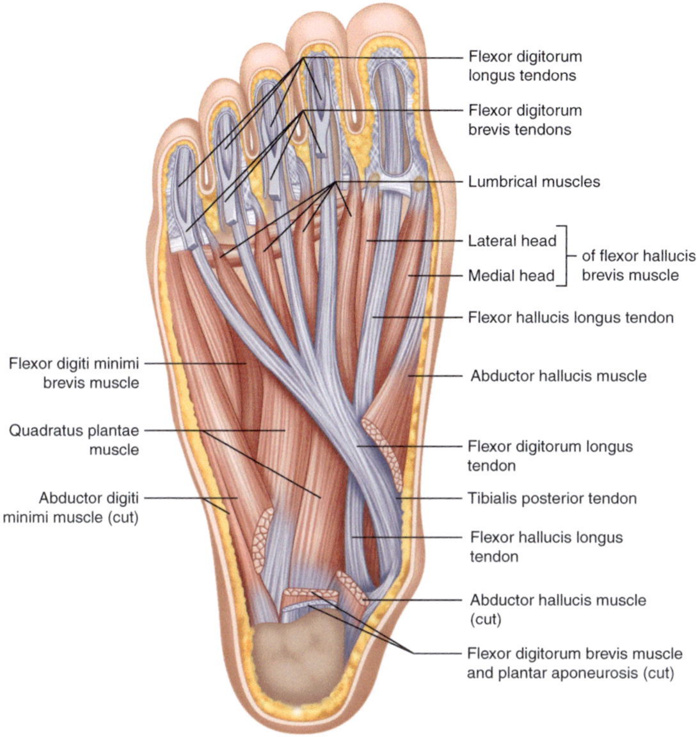

FIGURE 2.8 Muscles of sole of foot: second layer

The dorsalis pedis artery is the direct extension of the anterior tibial artery and travels between the tendons of extensor hallucis longus medially and extensor digitorum longus laterally. There are several important branches of dorsalis pedis artery to know

- a major terminal branch that travels deep in the 1st intermetatarsal space and joins the lateral plantar artery from the posterior tibial artery to form the plantar arch
- 1st dorsal metatarsal artery – supplies the dorsal skin of the 1st and 2nd toes

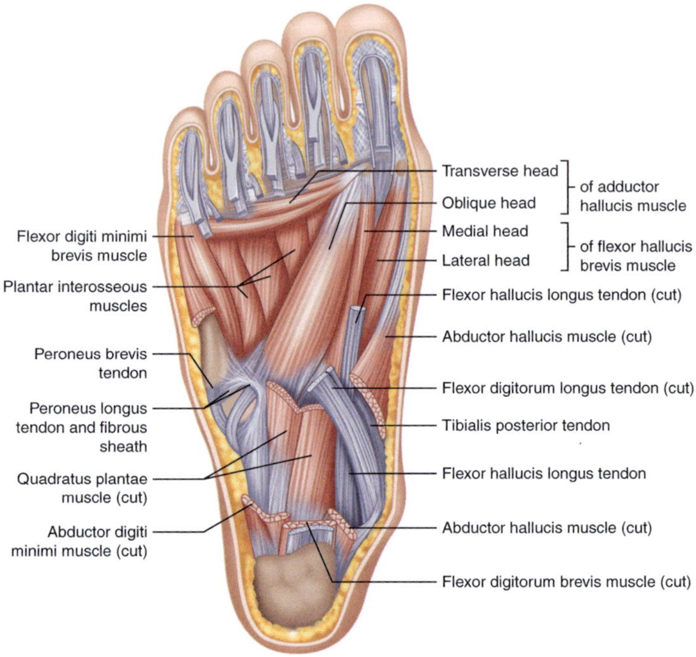

FIGURE 2.9 Muscles of sole of foot: third layer

- septocutaneous branches – supply the dorsal skin of the medial two-thirds of the foot which can be harvested as a fasciocutaneous flap based on dorsalis pedis artery

The medial and lateral plantar arteries are the terminal branches of the posterior tibial artery

- medial plantar artery – travels along the medial side of the foot and contributes to the plantar digital arteries of the 1st through 3rd digits
- lateral plantar artery – dominant blood supply of the plantar arch which provides blood supply to the toes via metatarsal branches

The terminal branches of the peroneal artery join with the lateral malleolar and calcaneal branches of the posterior tibial artery and mainly provide blood supply to the ankle.

Foot and Ankle Innervation

Motor innervation

- deep peroneal nerve – extensor hallucis brevis and extensor digitorum brevis
- tibial nerve – all the plantar intrinsic muscles via medial and lateral plantar branches

Cutaneous innervation

- sural nerve – lateral edge of foot via lateral calcaneal nerve
- saphenous nerve – medial edge of foot
- deep peroneal nerve – 1st web space
- superficial peroneal nerves – dorsal foot
- tibial nerve – sole of the foot via calcaneal, medial and lateral plantar branches

The Venous Anatomy of the Lower Extremity

The venous system of the lower extremity is divided into two groups, the deep veins and the superficial veins. The deep veins accompany their named arteries. There are two main superficial veins:

- the greater saphenous vein – originates at the medial aspect of the dorsal foot arch, ascends anterior to the medial malleolus, continues medially along the inner margin of the tibia posterior to the saphenous nerve, passes posteriorly to the medial femoral condyle and continues in the thigh to enter the femoral vein
- the lessor saphenous vein – originates at the lateral aspect of the dorsal foot arch, ascends posteriorly to the lateral malleolus, along the lateral aspect of the Achilles tendon, then runs medially to the posterior leg midline, perforates the deep fascia in the lower popliteal space and terminates in the popliteal vein

References

1. Boyer MI. AAOS comprehensive orthopaedic review, vol. 2. Rosemont: AAOS (American Academy of Orthopaedic Surgeons; 2014.
2. Neligan PC. Plastic surgery. London: Elsevier Saunders; 2018.
3. Netter FH. Atlas of human anatomy. Philadelphia: Elsevier; 2019.
4. Hansen JT. Netter's clinical anatomy. Amsterdam, The Netherlands: Elsevier; 2014.
5. Kaminsky AJ, Li SS, Copeland-Halperin LR, Miraliakbari R. The vastus lateralis free flap for lower extremity gustilo grade III reconstruction. Microsurgery. 2015;37:212–7.
6. Mujadzic T, Gober CA, Nahabedian DB, Ritter EF, Mujadzic M. Innervated pedicled gracilis flap for dynamic abdominal wall reconstruction. Plast Reconstr Surg Glob Open. 2018;6:e1852.
7. Lamaris GA, Carlisle MP, Durand P, Couto RA, Hendrickson MF. Maximizing the reach of the pedicled gastrocnemius muscle flap: a comparison of 2 surgical approaches. Ann Plast Surg. 2017;78:342–6.
8. Abou-Foul AK, Borumandi F. Anatomical variants of lower limb vasculature and implications for free fibula flap: systematic review and critical analysis. Microsurgery. 2015;36:165–72.
9. Ramanujam CL, Zgonis T. Use of local flaps for soft-tissue closure in diabetic foot wounds: a systematic review. Foot Ankle Spec. 2018:1938640018803745. https://doi.org/10.1177/1938640018803745. [Epub ahead of print].
10. Abdelrahman I, Elmasry M, Steinvall I, Olofsson P, Nettelblad H, Zdolsek J. Versatility of the extensor digitorum brevis muscle flap in lower limb reconstruction. Plast Reconstr Surg Glob Open. 2018;6:e2071.

Chapter 3
The Traumatized Leg

Rachel E. Hein, Rose Tillis, and Howard Levinson

Lower extremity trauma may result from motor vehicle collisions, falls, or accidents, and it often presents with multiple system involvement. Care begins with the initial trauma evaluation and stabilization. Multidisciplinary care is essential and typically involves trauma/critical care, plastic surgery, orthopedic surgery, and vascular surgery for the goal of limb salvage and prevention of complications.

R. E. Hein
Department of Surgery, Division of Plastic Surgery, Duke University Medical Center, Durham, NC, USA

R. Tillis
Division of Plastic Surgery, Duke University Hospital, Durham, NC, USA

H. Levinson (✉)
Departments of Surgery, Pathology, and Dermatology, Duke University Medical Center, Durham, NC, USA
e-mail: howard.levinson@duke.edu

S. T. Hollenbeck et al. (eds.), *Handbook of Lower Extremity Reconstruction*, https://doi.org/10.1007/978-3-030-41035-3_3

Acute Trauma Principles

Initial evaluation begins in the emergency department with established trauma protocols including Advanced Traumatic Life Support (ATLS) guidelines. Once the patient is stabilized (e.g. airway, breathing, circulation), a secondary survey begins. The secondary survey begins with inspection of open wounds and gross deformities. Documentation of wounds includes the degree of soft tissue injury, the presence of fractures, sensory and motor nerve injury, vascular compromise, and the presence of wound contamination [1]. If there are no overt signs of vascular injury, but injury is suspected, doppler examination of vessels and ankle brachial indexes (ABI) may be checked at the bedside (Fig. 3.1). An ABI <0.9 warrants additional evaluation. If there is high suspicion of vascular injury, imaging such as CT angiography or interventional angiography may be obtained, or the patient may proceed directly to the operating room.

Fractures are often present, and splinting may be used initially to stabilize the extremity, control bleeding, and minimize pain. Lower extremity fractures are most commonly classified according to the Gustilo classification system (Table 3.1). Classification variables include the size of the wound, the amount of soft tissue and bony injury, and the presence of vascular injury. Antibiotics covering gram-negative and gram-positive organisms should be started at the time of injury. For Gustilo type I and II injuries, antibiotics may be discontinued 24 hours after wound closure; for Gustilo type III injuries, antibiotics may be discontinued 72 hours after wound closure. In Gustilo type II and III wounds, a single dose of aminoglycosides at the time of injury is appropriate [2].

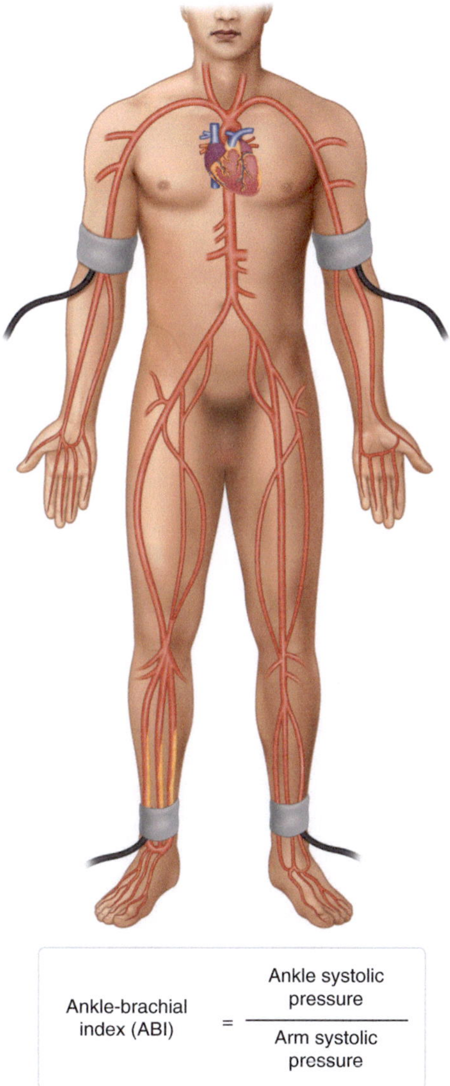

FIGURE 3.1 Diagram for assessing the ankle-brachial index (ABI). The ABI is determined by measuring the systolic blood pressures of the ankle and the ipsilateral arm and then dividing the ankle pressure by the arm pressure

TABLE 3.1 Gustilo classification of lower extremity injury

Grade	Details
I	Wound <1 cm Simple fracture, no comminution
II	Wound >1 cm Minimal soft tissue damage Moderate comminution/contamination
III	Extensive soft tissue damage, comminuted fracture, unstable
IIIA	Adequate soft tissue coverage
IIIB	Extensive soft tissue loss with periosteal stripping and exposed bone
IIIC	Arterial injury requiring repair

Adapted from Godina [12]; with permission

Compartment Pressure Evaluation and Treatment

Compartment pressure evaluation for limb ischemia is an important part of the initial evaluation. Compartment syndrome is a surgical disease, and acute compartment syndrome is a surgical emergency. It is caused by the build-up of pressure within a nonelastic muscle compartment where compartment pressure exceeds blood pressure; as a result, vascular perfusion is compromised. Compartment syndrome that is not treated within 6 hours of onset will lead to soft tissue infarct and extensive necrosis. In most instances, it is an avoidable disastrous complication of trauma.

There are four compartments in the lower extremity: anterior, lateral, superficial posterior, and deep posterior. Patients with crush injuries or vascular injuries, or those on anticoagulation are at an increased risk for compartment syndrome. Certain fracture patterns are at higher risk of compartment syndrome, including diaphyseal tibial fractures and tibial plateau fracture dislocations. There are several different approaches for assessing compartment pressures. The first is clinical examination, with special attention to the "5 P's"—pain, pallor, paralysis, paresthesia, and poikilothermia. Pain with passive stretch is the most sensitive physical exam finding and is often the first clinical sign of compartment syndrome. Compartmental pressures can be measured with a commercially available device or with a needle attached to an arterial line transducer. Compartment syndrome is diagnosed if the compartment pressure is greater than 30 mm Hg or if there is a difference between mean arterial pressure and the compartment pressure of less than 15 mm Hg. If there is any suspicion of compartment syndrome, the patient should be taken to the operating room immediately for compartment release. All four leg compartments are released via two skin incisions, which give access to the compartments (Fig. 3.2) [3].

Vascular and Orthopedic Intervention

Limb-threatening ischemia due to vascular injury is another condition that requires rapid identification and treatment. Penetrating trauma with obvious vascular injury should be addressed in the operating room immediately via direct vessel repair, shunt, or bypass. Ischemia time greater than 3 to 4 hours may lead to limb death, so vascular repair will supersede orthopedic repair as needed and often includes limb fasciotomies.

Orthopedic fixation is performed using a variety of methods, including external fixators, intramedullary nails, or plates, depending on the injury. Débridement is typically performed prior to or at the time of orthopedic fixation and must be comprehensive. Punctate bone bleeding ("the paprika sign") is a sign of healthy tissue and indicates a reduced risk of nonunion and osteomyelitis [4].

Leg fasciotomy

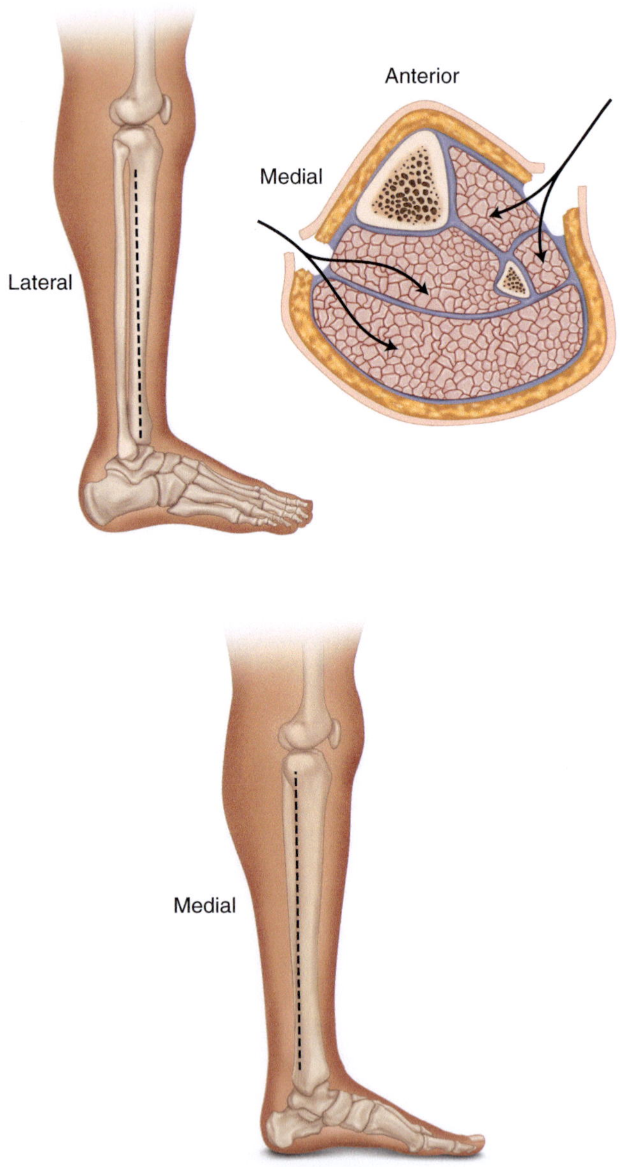

FIGURE 3.2 Incision placement for lower extremity compartment release. There are two skin incisions—one medial and one lateral—and four fasciotomy incisions. The lateral skin incision provides access to the anterior and lateral compartments. The medial skin incision provides access to the deep and superficial posterior compartments [3]. *Black broken line* indicates the incision line for a one-incision technique for release of medial and lateral compartments

Osteomyelitis

The risk of osteomyelitis in lower extremity trauma occurs in up to 8% of patients, according to the LEAP study [5]. The tibia is the most common site for non-union and osteomyelitis. The most common pathogen in osteomyelitis is *Staphylococcus aureus* or multiorganism infections including *Pseudomonas aeruginosa*. Risk factors for major infections include Gustilo IIIC tibial fractures, segmental bone loss greater than 2 cm, delayed presentation, and use of an external fixator. Timing of débridement or degree of contamination has not been shown to increase infection rates. If osteomyelitis is suspected, common diagnostic modalities include MRI imaging and laboratory tests (white blood cell count, erythrocyte sedimentation rate, and c-reactive protein). The gold standard for diagnosis is bone biopsy.

Treatment is critically important, as osteomyelitis often leads to malunion, chronic pain, and limb loss. Treatment typically involves a multidisciplinary team including orthopedics, infectious disease, and plastic surgery, and it typically includes serial wide débridement, fracture stabilization, possible placement of antibiotic-impregnated cement, and at least 6 weeks of intravenous antibiotics [5–7].

Deciding Between Limb Amputation vs. Salvage

Several studies have attempted to delineate trauma patients that would benefit from amputation versus limb salvage. The first of these studies produced the Mangled Extremity

Table 3.2 Mangled extremity severity score

Variable	Score
A. Skeletal and Soft Tissue Injury	
Low energy (stable, simple fracture, civilian gunshot wound)	1
Medium energy (open/multiple fractures, dislocation)	2
High energy (close-range shotgun, military gunshot wound, crush)	3
Very high energy (above + gross contamination)	4
B. Limb Ischemia	
Pulse reduced or absent; perfusion normal	1
Pulseless, paresthesias, diminished capillary refill	2
Cool, paralyzed, insensate, numb	3
C. Shock	
Systolic blood pressure > 90 mm Hg	1
Transient hypotension	2
Persistent hypotension	3
D. Age	
<30 years	1
30–50 years	2
>50 years	3
Threshold Score for Amputation	**7**

Adapted from Johansen [8]; with permission

Severity Score (Table 3.2), which was based on skeletal and soft tissue injury, limb ischemia, shock, and patient age. A score of 7 or greater was used as a threshold to determine patients who should have an amputation [8]. This approach was met with controversy, so a second approach to evaluate salvage potential was proposed in the LEAP (Lower Extremity Assessment Project) study. Results from the

LEAP study revealed that patients with severe extremity trauma tend to come from lower socioeconomic backgrounds, but the study failed to describe definitive criteria for determining which patients would benefit from amputation versus limb salvage [9]. The generally accepted factors that lead surgeons and patients to choose amputation over limb salvage include Gustilo IIIC injury, sciatic or tibial nerve injury, prolonged ischemia time (>6 hours), crush or significant soft tissue injury, significant wound contamination, multiple comminuted fractures or segmental bone fractures, increasing age or severe comorbidities, low social support system, and finally, failed revascularization [8, 9]. If amputation is deemed necessary, one should preserve as much limb length as feasible. Below-knee amputations have been shown to require less energy demand for ambulation than above-knee amputations, so preserving limb length is valuable [10, 11].

Timing of Reconstruction

Once the patient has been stabilized and orthopedic and vascular injuries have been managed, soft tissue reconstructive planning begins. Planning includes consideration of patient comorbidities such as concomitant injuries (e.g., head trauma with intracranial bleeding), organ failure, tobacco use, or cardiac disease; patient age; baseline functional status; and patient wishes. In a landmark study in 1986, Godina reported that immediate extremity reconstruction within 72 hours of injury had the lowest incidence of complications and the best outcomes [12] (Table 3.3). Shortcomings of this study included non-randomization of patients, variable reconstructions, inclusion of both upper and lower extremity trauma, and initial treatment delay of the first 100 patients. Several supporting and refuting articles have been published since Godina's original study, and negative pressure wound therapy (NPWT) has also gained in popularity [5, 6, 12]. While early reconstruction is accepted, some injuries may not be amena-

Table 3.3 Godina's results on timing of microsurgical repair

	Timing of repair		
Variable	**Early (<72 h)**	**Delayed (72 h–3 mo)**	**Late (>3 mo)**
Number of patients	134	167	231
Free flap failures	0.75%	12%	22%
Postoperative infection	1.5%	17.5%	6%
Bone healing time, months	6.8 mo	12.3 mo	29 mo
Time in hospital (average)	27 days	130 days	256 days
Number of surgeries (average)	1.3	4.1	7.8

Adapted from Godina [12]; with permission

ble to early treatment, and NPWT may be used for late-stage reconstruction. NPWT has been shown to decrease the need for flap reconstruction [13].

Complications and Pitfalls

Common complications of lower extremity salvage include limb loss, hemorrhage, rhabdomyolysis, osteomyelitis, nonunion, and deep venous thrombosis or venous thromboembolism (VTE) [14]. Acute uncontrolled hemorrhage is the second leading cause of death after injury. Bleeding should be immediately assessed, controlled, and aggressively treated following the ATLS protocol. VTE is also a serious and preventable cause of death, although it generally presents 21 to 24 days after injury [15]. VTE is prevented and treated with anticoagulation based on the patient's renal function, weight, and comorbid conditions. Common prophylactic anticoagulation includes unfractionated heparin (5000 U three times daily) or enoxaparin (Lovenox®) 40 mg daily or 30 mg twice daily. Another complication in lower extremity injury is rhabdomyolysis associated with crush mechanisms. Rhabdomyolysis may lead to renal failure and death, and volume replacement is key in treatment. Finally, bony non-union is the most common long-term complication of lower extremity trauma (up to 24%) [15].

Conclusion

Overall, lower extremity trauma is a major cause of morbidity with many social implications. Initial treatment should focus on stabilization of the patient, followed by addressing secondary injuries and preventing complications. Gustilo IIIC tibial fractures have the worst prognosis. Treatment should include an experienced multidisciplinary team because decision making and treatments can be complex.

References

1. Gustilo RB, Mendoza RM, Williams DN. Problems in the management of type III (severe) open fractures: a new classification of type III open fractures. J Trauma. 1984;24:742–6.
2. Gustilo RB. Management of open fractures and complications. Instr Course Lect. 1982;31:64–75.
3. Schmidt AH. Acute compartment syndrome. Orthop Clin North Am. 2016;47:517–25.
4. Ong YS, Levin LS. Lower limb salvage in trauma. Plast Reconstr Surg. 2010;125:582–8.
5. Pollak AN, Jones AL, Castillo RC, Bosse MJ, MacKenzie EJ, LEAP Study Group. The relationship between time to surgical débridement and incidence of infection after open high-energy lower extremity trauma. J Bone Joint Surg Am. 2010;92:7–15.
6. Francel TJ, Vander Kolk CA, Hoopes JE, Manson PN, Yaremchuk MJ. Microvascular soft-tissue transplantation for reconstruction of acute open tibial fractures: timing of coverage and long-term functional results. Plast Reconstr Surg. 1992;89:478–87; discussion 488–9.

7. Butcher JL, MacKenzie EJ, Cushing B, Jurkovich G, Morris J, Burgess A, et al. Long-term outcomes after lower extremity trauma. J Trauma. 1996;41:4–9.
8. Johansen K, Daines M, Howey T, Helfet D, Hansen ST Jr. Objective criteria accurately predict amputation following lower extremity trauma. J Trauma. 1990;30:568–72; discussion 572–3.
9. Higgins TF, Klatt JB, Beals TC. Lower Extremity Assessment Project (LEAP)--the best available evidence on limb-threatening lower extremity trauma. Orthop Clin North Am. 2010;41:233–9.
10. Bosse MJ, McCarthy ML, Jones AL, Webb LX, Sims SH, Sanders RW, MacKenzie EJ, Lower Extremity Assessment Project (LEAP) Study Group. The insensate foot following severe lower extremity trauma: an indication for amputation? J Bone Joint Surg Am. 2005;87:2601–8.
11. MacKenzie EJ, Bosse MJ, Castillo RC, Smith DG, Webb LX, Kellam JF, et al. Functional outcomes following trauma-related lower-extremity amputation. J Bone Joint Surg Am. 2004;86-A:1636–45.
12. Godina M. Early microsurgical reconstruction of complex trauma of the extremities. Plast Reconstr Surg. 1986;78:285–92.
13. Kolker AR, Kasabian AK, Karp NS, Gottlieb JJ. Fate of free flap microanastomosis distal to the zone of injury in lower extremity trauma. Plast Reconstr Surg. 1997;99:1068–73.
14. Pollak AN, McCarthy ML, Burgess AR. Short-term wound complications after application of flaps for coverage of traumatic soft-tissue defects about the tibia. The Lower Extremity Assessment Project (LEAP) Study Group. J Bone Joint Surg Am. 2000;82-A:1681–91.
15. Arcelus JI, Monreal M, Caprini JA, Guisado JG, Soto MJ, Núñez MJ, Alvárez JC. RIETE investigators. Clinical presentation and time-course of postoperative venous thromboembolism: results from the RIETE registry. Thromb Haemost. 2008;99:546–51.

Chapter 4
Orthopaedic Principles of Lower Extremity Injuries

Lily R. Mundy, Daniel J. Cunningham, and Mark J. Gage

Fracture management, the biology of bone healing, and the physiologic implications of extremity injuries are all equally important factors that should be considered together. Fractures do not occur in isolation and are associated with concomitant soft tissue injuries of varying degrees. Treatment should be properly planned so that fracture management occurs in concert with management of other injuries to facilitate early mobilization and optimize the ultimate function of the injured extremity.

Fracture Fixation

There are several fracture immobilization strategies that vary in level of invasiveness for the patient. Casting and splinting are least invasive, but they often prohibit mobilization of the

L. R. Mundy
Division of Plastic and Reconstructive Surgery, Duke University, Durham, NC, USA

D. J. Cunningham · M. J. Gage (✉)
Department of Orthopaedic Surgery, Duke University, Durham, NC, USA
e-mail: mark.gage@duke.edu

S. T. Hollenbeck et al. (eds.), *Handbook of Lower Extremity Reconstruction*, https://doi.org/10.1007/978-3-030-41035-3_4

affected extremity. External fixation and internal fixation allow for better fracture control with direct immobilization, and they often facilitate earlier mobilization of that extremity. The anatomic goal of fracture fixation is to restore length, alignment, and rotation, whereas the functional goal of fracture fixation is to provide an appropriate biomechanical environment for healing and patient mobilization. The choice of a fracture fixation construct is sometimes complex and often depends on balancing factors affecting fracture healing with patient-specific and fracture-specific needs.

One factor that plays a large role in selecting a fixation strategy is the degree of bony comminution induced by the forces involved in the injury. Comminuted fractures have many pieces that cannot reasonably be placed precisely back into their original location without causing considerable additional injury to the bone and surrounding blood supply. On the other hand, simple fractures involve few pieces that often can be brought back to their original location and fixed.

A second determinant of fracture fixation strategy is the anatomic location of the fracture. For fractures involving the diaphysis, or long tubular portion of bone, there is less emphasis placed on ensuring precise realignment of individual fracture fragments. Rather, the overall length, alignment, and rotation of the bone should be restored. In contrast, fractures involving the articular surface receive special attention, and great care is taken to restore individual fracture fragments to their original anatomic location in order to re-create smooth joint surfaces, to avoid cartilage wear that may be related to the development of arthritis. In general, fracture gaps greater than 2 mm are not tolerated.

A third determinant of fracture fixation strategy is the desired type of bony healing. Two types of stability are achieved with fracture fixation: absolute and relative stability. These two types of fixation are defined by the degree of "strain" or fracture motion that is allowed. Absolute stability reduces the strain between fracture fragments through rigid and precise immobilization of these fracture fragments, using methods such as application of specific types of plates and screws. This fixation method is important in peri-articular fractures and some simple long bone diaphyseal fractures. Conversely, relative stability allows greater strain between fragments, using methods such as casting, splinting, bracing, external fixation, intramedullary fixation, and application of special types of bridging plates and screws. The following are examples of each type of fracture fixation.

Casting, *splinting*, and *bracing* are fracture fixation methods that keep fractures reduced through pressure exerted by the material onto the soft tissues surrounding the bone. These methods are appropriate treatments for many fractures. In the lower extremity, they are helpful in providing initial stabilization, reduction, and pain control prior to definitive fixation, and they may be appropriate definitive treatment for fractures that are nondisplaced or minimally displaced. Close follow-up with an orthopaedic surgeon is important to ensure that these fractures do not displace. If they do, operative treatment may be indicated to achieve the most functional outcome.

External fixation is a fracture fixation method that involves percutaneously applied pins that transfix fracture fragments, which are then fixed to an external frame. This fracture fixation method can be applied relatively quickly and is minimally invasive. This method of fracture fixation does not often achieve precise anatomic reduction; it is indicated for situations in which operative time is limited due to patient and environmental factors and/or in which a soft tissue injury or infection precludes definitive internal fixation. Examples of fractures appropriate for initial external fixation include high-energy peri-articular fractures of the knee and ankle, as well as diaphyseal fractures of the femur and tibia in the polytraumatized patient. In general, patients with external fixators are kept non-weightbearing on the operative extremity until fracture union or definitive internal fixation. Because the pins pass through the skin into bone, it is critical to ensure that these areas are routinely cleaned.

Perhaps the most recognizable form of fracture fixation is *internal fixation* with plates, screws, and/or intramedullary devices. Fixation with intramedullary devices is most often applied to simple and comminuted diaphyseal fractures of the femur and tibia, in which precise reduction of individual fracture fragments is not critical. In the case of fracture fixation with an intramedullary device, the fracture is often reduced through closed means, and a rod or "nail" is passed through the intramedullary canal. This nail can then be transfixed at one or both ends with screws that lock the proximal and distal aspects of the fractured bone, setting the extremity's length, alignment, and rotation. Intramedullary fixation often allows immediate weightbearing on the affected extremity. On the other hand, fractures requiring precise fragment realignment, such as peri-articular fractures, often undergo open reduction followed by fixation with plates and screws that are contoured to the patient's anatomy. In general, patients have restricted weightbearing after fixation with plates and screws because it is important to maintain the reduction that was achieved at the time of the operation. During the operation, great care is taken to avoid further damaging the often-tenuous blood supply of the fractured bones and the surrounding tissues, in order to facilitate fracture healing. New advances in minimally invasive reduction and fixation techniques are minimizing the soft tissue damage caused by open reduction and fixation.

Osseous Healing

Fracture fixation methods affect the type of osseous healing that takes place. There are two types of bony healing, which are termed primary and secondary. Relative stability, which allows more strain than absolute stability, typically achieves secondary or "indirect" bone healing. In this type of osseous healing, there is a progression from fracture hematoma to soft callus to hard callus, and, eventually, to remodeled bone. Specifically, the initial fracture hematoma contains progenitor cells that differentiate into cells such as osteoblasts and chondrocytes, which are critical for fracture healing. These cells then form the soft callus through production of osteoid (bone matrix) and/or cartilage. Soft callus is converted to a calcified cartilage matrix or hard callus, which is then further developed into mechanically acceptable bone through remodeling by osteoclasts and osteoblasts.

In contrast to relative stability, absolute stability, which induces a low-strain environment, allows primary or "direct" bone healing. Direct bone healing is the process of direct bone formation without the need for a cartilaginous intermediate scaffold. In this type of healing, the osteoclasts and osteoblasts pass through the fracture site and sequentially resorb and deposit new bone. In reality, these types of bone healing may co-exist in fractures, but it is important for the surgeon to anticipate the type of osseous healing achieved by the fixation construct that will be applied.

External Fixation in the Setting of Acute Trauma

External fixation is a particularly appropriate initial stabilization strategy for patients with acute, life-threatening trauma. External fixation can be rapidly applied to achieve an initial reduction, which can help with pain control and fracture bleeding. Additionally, external fixation causes minimal additional soft tissue injury, and pre-existing soft tissue injuries can be accessed in ways that are not possible with casting and splinting. Lastly, external fixation avoids the concern for increased systemic inflammation and pulmonary injury that is potentially induced by intramedullary nailing of lower extremity fractures through embolization of intramedullary contents to the lungs. External fixators may be used for definitive treatment of fractures, but they have limitations in terms of weightbearing and anatomic reduction. For this reason, patients with external fixators may often be transitioned to definitive internal fixation once their soft tissue and medical status allows.

Bone Loss after Trauma

In the setting of bone loss, it is important to evaluate the anatomic location, condition, and vascularity of the surrounding soft tissues, in addition to the size and character of the bone defect. A large-segment osseous defect, or fractures without an intact, well-vascularized soft tissue envelope, may not heal with adequate stabilization of the fracture segments alone. These are termed "critical defects" and often require additional interventions. These defects are typically associated with significant soft tissue injury resulting in a relatively dysvascular boney injury with low healing potential. Treatments considered for these bone defects are largely contingent on their size. Small osseous critical defects are typically effectively managed by bone grafting, whereas larger defects are more commonly treated with distraction osteogenesis or the induced membrane technique. Vascularized bone free-tissue transfer also may play a role in lower extremity trauma.

Bone Reconstruction: Small-Scale Defects

The ideal bone grafting material will have three key properties of bone remodeling: osteogenesis, osteoinduction, and osteoconduction. *Osteogenesis* describes natural bone growth; an osteogenic graft will have viable osteoprogenitor cells within the graft material. *Osteoinduction* is the ability to induce surrounding undifferentiated and pluripotent cells into osteoblasts, or bone cells. *Osteoconduction* describes the presence of the scaffold onto which new bone grows. Lastly, *osteointegration* describes the creation of a structural and functional union between bone and a prosthetic material.

Autologous bone is the gold standard for bone graft. It is most commonly harvested from the iliac crest of the pelvis. As shown on Table 4.1, autologous bone possesses osteogenic, osteoinductive, and osteoconductive properties with no risk of disease transmission. Its drawbacks, however, are the potential for donor site morbidity, such as pain and infection,

Table 4.1 Bone remodeling properties of bone graft

	Osteogenesis	Osteoinduction	Osteoconduction
Autologous bone	X	X	X
Allograft bone		X (variable)	X
Calcium phosphates and calcium sulfates			X

Table 4.2 Autologous bone harvest sites and associated graft volumes

Autologous bone harvest site	Graft volume
Posterior iliac crest	60–80 cc
Anterior iliac crest	40–60 cc
Proximal femur	30–40 cc
Distal femur	30–50 cc
Proximal tibia	30–50 cc
Distal tibia	15–20 cc
Calcaneus	10–15 cc

as well as the potential limitations in the quantity that can be harvested (Table 4.2).

In addition to traditional methods of bone graft harvest, intramedullary graft can be harvested through a reamer device that collects bone as it is advanced through the intramedullary canal. This allows for large bone graft volumes (40–60 cc) with faster harvest time, lower postoperative pain scores, and decreased complications when compared with iliac crest bone harvest. However, using this technique for intramedullary bone collection has its associated implant costs due to the device needed to harvest [1]. Alternatives to autologous bone grafting for small defects include allograft, demineralized bone matrix, and calcium phosphates and calcium sulfates. Allograft bone and calcium sulfates/phosphates have osteoconductive and in some cases limited osteoinductive properties. Additionally, they avoid the donor site morbidity concerns that occur with autograft. However, allograft has a potential for disease transmission, and both come at a significant implant cost.

Bone Reconstruction: Large-Scale Defects

There are two primary methods of reconstruction of large osseous defects: the induced membrane technique and distraction osteogenesis. The induced-membrane technique is a two-stage process that was first described by Alain Masquelet and colleagues [2]. The first stage includes débridement of the defect site and placement of a cement spacer. This cement spacer induces a foreign-body reaction, resulting in the formation of a membrane (Fig. 4.1) that has favorable character-

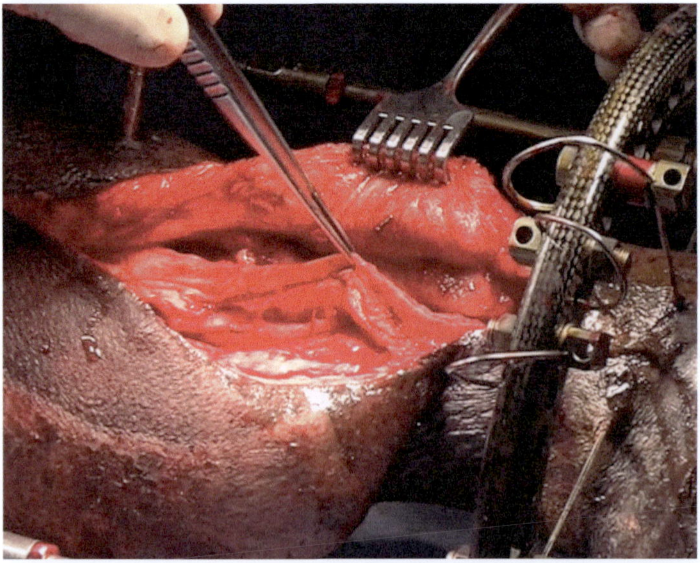

FIGURE 4.1 Example of a membrane being formed for use in the induced-membrane technique for reconstruction of bone defects

istics for bone regeneration. During the second stage, the cement spacer is explanted, taking care to preserve the encapsulating membrane. The residual space within the membrane is then bone grafted, and the membrane is closed over the graft. Membrane characteristics change over time, with the most favorable characteristics of the membrane for bone regeneration peaking at approximately 4–8 weeks [2].

Distraction osteogenesis is the second technique commonly used for large defects. This technique treats bone defects by taking a bone segment that is cut and translating it through the defect. The site of distraction will fill in with bone and the translated segment slowly closes down the defect (Fig. 4.2) until union is reached. An alternative method with this technique is to acutely shorten the limb across the bone defect and then distract the limb over time to the appropriate length. This may be a preferable option to reduce tension on a wound closure or simplify a soft tissue defect.

The induced-membrane technique augments local biology by increasing the local level of growth factors. The membrane prevents graft resorption, and the technique can be a useful tool in contaminated wounds, as bone grafting is delayed, allowing for adequate time to observe the soft tissue envelope. However, bone consolidation rates are less consistent with this technique, and multiple operations are required. Time to union has ranged from 6.2 to 14.4 months, and union success rates have been 82–90%, with an average of four to six surgeries [3, 4]. Distraction osteogenesis leads to more consistent bone production and can obviate the need for complex soft tissue reconstruction with shortening, but this technique is demanding for the surgeon and the patient, requiring frequent follow-up and a reliable patient. It also has higher complication rates. Time to union has ranged from 12.2 to 15.8 months, with 92% union success rates [5, 6].

Vascularized autograft is frequently used for large-segment bone reconstruction of the upper extremity and mandible/maxilla, but it also can have a role in the lower extremity. Vascularized autograft in lower extremity segmental bone loss is associated with union rates of 87–98%. The primary limitation with this technique is that the vascularized graft

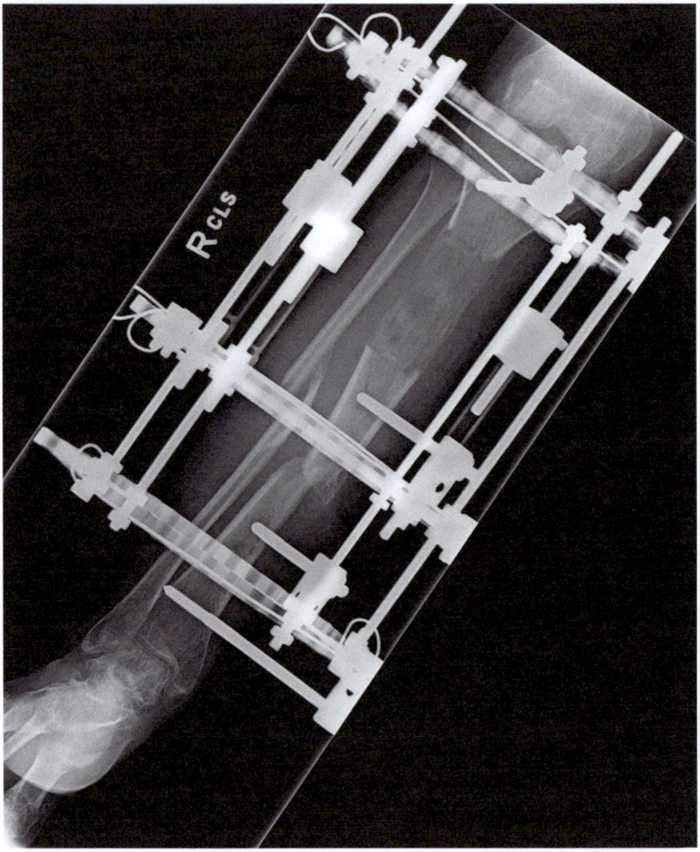

FIGURE 4.2 An example of distraction osteogenesis in the treatment of a segmental tibia defect after open fracture. Note the regenerate bone being formed in the proximal tibia as the middle tibial segment is being translated distally to fill the defect

does not match the cortical width of the femur or tibia, and because of this mismatch in caliber, it can fracture with physiologic loads over time. The reported 2-year fracture rate is 15–40% [7, 8]. For this reason, vascularized bone autograft is not frequently utilized by lower extremity reconstructive surgeons.

Summary

Lower extremity fractures should not be considered in isolation, but rather as a key component in the reconstruction process. Restoring skeletal stability should occur early in this process, to serve as a foundation for further reconstructive efforts and to facilitate early patient mobilization. Definitive reconstruction may require more than fracture fixation alone when bone loss has occurred. The techniques employed to achieve bone union are predicated on the injury's characteristics and patient factors.

References

1. Dawson J, Kiner D, Gardner W 2nd, Swafford R, Nowotarski PJ. The reamer-irrigator-aspirator as a device for harvesting bone graft compared with iliac crest bone graft: union rates and complications. J Orthop Trauma. 2014;28:584–90.
2. Pelissier P, Masquelet AC, Bareille R, Pelissier SM, Amedee J. Induced membranes secrete growth factors including vascular and osteoinductive factors and could stimulate bone regeneration. J Orthop Res. 2004;22:73–9.
3. Taylor BC, Hancock J, Zitzke R, Castaneda J. Treatment of bone loss with the induced membrane technique: techniques and outcomes. J Orthop Trauma. 2015;29:554–7.
4. Karger C, Kishi T, Schneider L, Fitoussi F, Masquelet AC. French Society of Orthopaedic Surgery and Traumatology (SoFCOT). Treatment of posttraumatic bone defects by the induced membrane technique. Orthop Traumatol Surg Res. 2012;98:97–102.
5. Mekhail AO, Abraham E, Gruber B, Gonzalez M. Bone transport in the management of posttraumatic bone defects in the lower extremity. J Trauma. 2004;56:368–78.
6. Oh CW, Song HR, Roh JY, Oh JK, Min WK, Kyung HS, et al. Bone transport over an intramedullary nail for reconstruction of long bone defects in tibia. Arch Orthop Trauma Surg. 2008;128:801–8.
7. Song HR, Kale A, Park HB, Koo KH, Chae DJ, Oh CW, Chung DW. Comparison of internal bone transport and vascularized fibular grafting for femoral bone defects. J Orthop Trauma. 2003;17:203–11.
8. Yazar S, Lin CH, Wei FC. One-stage reconstruction of composite bone and soft-tissue defects in traumatic lower extremities. Plast Reconstr Surg. 2004;114:1457–66.

Chapter 5
Reconstruction of Oncologic Defects

Franca Kraenzlin and Justin M. Sacks

General Principles

A wide array of benign and malignant tumors can affect the lower extremities, from benign soft tissue tumors to osteosarcomas, soft tissue sarcomas, and cutaneous malignancies [1, 2]. The reconstructive surgeon is frequently called upon to close large defects spanning multiple tissue layers. Historically, limb amputation was the standard of care, but new therapies and reconstructive advances have ushered in an era of limb salvage. Restoration of form and function remains the most basic reconstructive principle applied to the patient requiring oncologic resection, and it is especially important in the lower extremity, given the goal of painless ambulation following recovery.

While all rungs of the reconstructive ladder can be utilized, special circumstances affecting the cancer patient must be considered [3]. The health of a cancer patient is an important

F. Kraenzlin
Department of Plastic Surgery, Johns Hopkins Hospital, Owings Mills, MD, USA

J. M. Sacks (✉)
Department of Plastic and Reconstructive Surgery, Johns Hopkins School of Medicine, Baltimore, MD, USA

S. T. Hollenbeck et al. (eds.), *Handbook of Lower Extremity Reconstruction*, https://doi.org/10.1007/978-3-030-41035-3_5

consideration in operative planning. Nutrition labs, an analysis of weight change, and functional status are all important components of the pre-operative evaluation. A patient's ability to tolerate a lengthy surgery, bleeding, prolonged immobility, and the known complications of reconstructive procedures need to be considered prior to creating a surgical plan. The oncologic goal, whether to obtain disease-free margins or to perform a palliative resection, must be known, and the ideal timing between surgery and further cancer therapies should also be considered before developing a plan for surgery that may have a prolonged recovery time.

Reconstructive timing needs to be considered, especially when microscopically margin-negative resection (R0) is desired. Immediate reconstruction is generally considered the preferred technique, as tissue planes are readily visible, but delayed reconstruction may be necessary if margin status cannot be established. If a delayed reconstructive procedure is necessary, the surgeon should prepare the wound bed for reconstruction and specify preferred dressings until definitive reconstruction can be performed. Though simple wound closures can be performed with unknown margin status, larger surgeries such as tissue expansion and microvascular free tissue transfer should not be performed without such knowledge.

The oncologic and reconstructive surgeons should discuss the possible structures to be resected. Advanced imaging can show tumor dimensions, abutting structures, and infiltrated structures with detail, allowing for preoperative assessment of the complexity of resection. When it comes to tumor removal, four different types of resection are possible (Fig. 5.1). Intralesional resections occur when the surgeon enters the tumor at any point during the surgery and resects portions of the tumor, aiming either for a debulking procedure or relying on subsequent therapies to eliminate macroscopic disease. Marginal resections remove the tumor along its pseudo-capsule within the reactive tissue plane, whereas a wide resection encompasses tumor and the reactive zone, dissecting entirely through normal tissue. Finally, a radical excision includes removal of the tumor, the pseudo-capsule, and the entire involved myofascial or bony compartment.

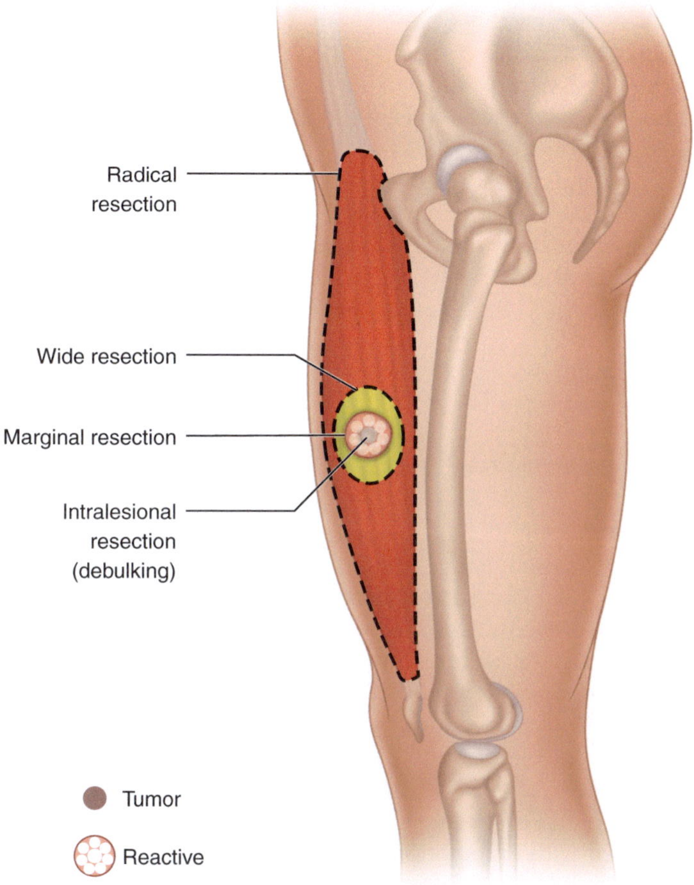

FIGURE 5.1 Types of sarcoma tumor resections include intralesional resection, marginal resection, wide resection (*yellow*), and radical resection (*red*)

Depending on the tumor location and resection type, removal could involve bone, major vessels, nerves, muscle groups, and overlying skin, all of which will require repair when performing an adequate reconstruction. Prior knowledge of the type of resection necessary can ensure adequate selection of biomaterials, donor sites, dressings, and postoperative therapies, while also providing the patient with foresight about the extent of recovery.

Finally, the possibility of adjuvant or neoadjuvant radiation must always be considered by the reconstructive surgeon. Tension-free repairs and vascularized tissue are required to withstand the scourges of radiation therapy; skin grafts should necessarily be avoided.

Massive osteocutaneous defects requiring reconstruction of bony and soft tissue components can occur during limb salvage surgery. As a result, the importance of careful planning and collaboration with the oncologic surgeon cannot be understated.

Bony Reconstruction

There are a number of malignant and benign primary bone tumors that, though rare, require resection of large segments of bony tissues. Osteosarcomas are the most common primary malignant bone tumors and are generally treated with a combination of surgical resection and chemotherapy [4]. Survival historically was as low as 10% at 5 years, but advances in imaging, chemotherapy, and reconstructive techniques have improved that figure to 66–82%. More than 90% of patients undergo limb salvage, which has a slightly higher rate of local recurrence but no negative impact on long-term survival when compared with amputation. Resection of osteosarcomas typically includes 2 cm of normal tissue, and osteotomies are generally performed with a cuff of 3–5 cm of normal bone.

Bony reconstruction is typically performed by the oncologic orthopedic surgeon, as most bone tumors occur in the metaphyseal portion of long bones, generally requiring resection of the entire proximal or distal portion of the bone with its joint. Insertion of a prosthesis is then required, efficiently replacing large segments of bones and the corresponding removed joints. Expandable prostheses now allow for noninvasive limb lengthening for young patients, but reattachment of tendons and long-term breakage of the device remain problematic.

However, intercalary resections are frequently possible, especially when tumors include the diaphyseal portion of a bone. Intercalary resections remove segments of bone while maintaining the native joints, achieving better functional outcomes than an endoprosthetic. There are a number of reconstructive options for intercalary defects, including allografts, devitalized autografts, intercalary prosthetics, and bone transport using an external fixator. Uses of devitalized autografts or allografts have shown high rates of complications, including fracture, infection, and nonunion. A segmental prosthesis allows high rates of adequate postoperative functioning, but the benefits are short-term, with roughly 37% of prostheses failing by the 10-year mark [5, 6]. Bone transport allows for reconstruction of large bony defects and eliminates donor site morbidity, but at a cost of a labor-intensive, lengthy, and uncomfortable process. Composite grafts using vascularized fibula grafts and devitalized autografts or allografts can reliably be used to overcome the complications of fracture, infection, and nonunion that plague some of the other reconstructive techniques, providing a reconstruction lasting a lifetime (Fig. 5.2).

Soft Tissue Reconstruction

Once bony stability has been achieved, the surgeon must reconstruct the soft tissue of the lower extremity. Planning should account for muscular, arterial, nerve, adipose, and cutaneous tissue resections. Osteosarcomas often require soft tissue resection, but isolated soft tissue tumors can also occur.

Soft tissue sarcomas are complicated tumors of connecting tissue that typically present as a painless mass and traditionally required limb amputation. As with bony tumors, however, studies have shown that individuals undergoing limb-sparing resection and radiotherapy, though having higher rates of local recurrence than with amputation, had no differences in rates of disease-free survival or overall survival at 5 years. As a result, limb salvage is now the preferred method of tumor resection [1, 2, 4].

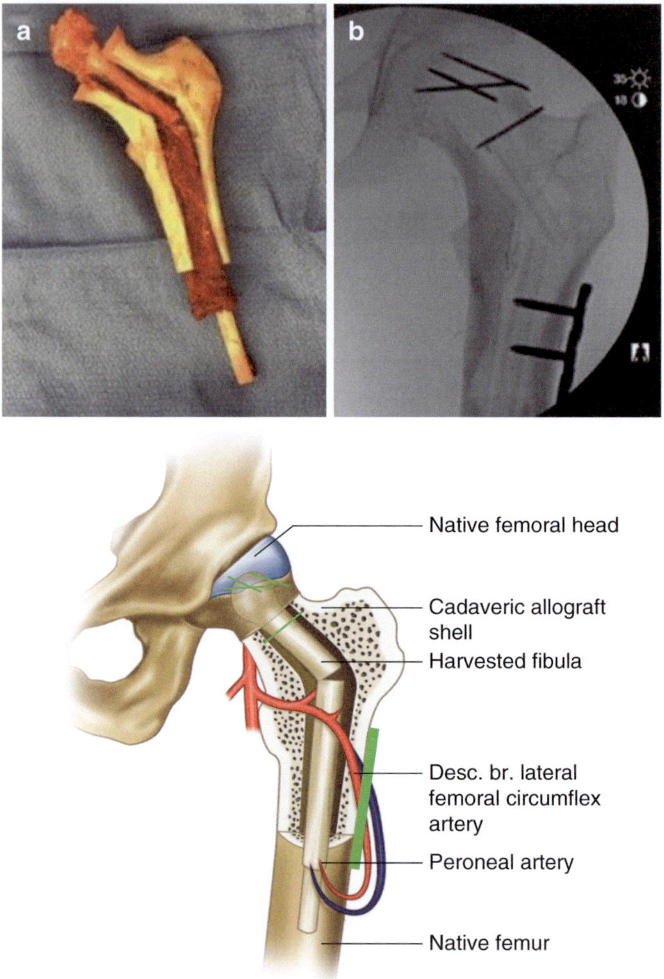

Figure 5.2 Composite vascularized autograft for reconstruction of an intercalary defect involving the hip joint. (**a**) This allograft hip has been fitted with an internal vascularized fibula bone flap. (**b**) The hip construct has been placed into the patient. The fluoroscopy image demonstrates a plate and several pins securing the fibula bone flap in position within the allograft. The schematic of the construct, shown for clarity, includes the vascularization with the descending branch (desc. br.) of the lateral femoral circumflex artery and the peroneal artery

Biopsy is typically performed to establish a histologic diagnosis and grade of the tumor (based on cell differentiation, mitotic count, and necrosis), to assist with surgical planning and adjunctive therapies. The extent of resection to obtain negative margins and minimize local recurrence is typically 1 cm, save for specific considerations given to certain sarcoma subtypes. Microscopic positive margins (R1 resection) following tumor resection does not subsequently guarantee local recurrence, so critical vascular or nerve structures usually are not sacrificed to obtain an R0 resection.

There is clear evidence that radiation reduces the risk of local recurrence without impacting disease-free survival. Therefore, radiation is recommended most strongly for patients with large (≥5 cm), high-grade sarcomas with significant risk of local recurrence. Though radiation can be administered as either adjuvant or neoadjuvant therapy without differences in long-term survival or recurrence, complication rates do differ. Patients undergoing neoadjuvant radiation therapy are more likely to require reoperation and have wound complications, whereas those receiving adjuvant therapy have been more likely to suffer from joint fibrosis.

Rates of local recurrence are approximately 40% to 60%, but the timing of recurrence differs by grade. High-grade tumors typically all recur within 5 years, with over 50% recurring within the first 2 years. Low-grade tumors recur later, with roughly half recurring more than 5 years after resection. Allowances should always be made for the possibility of reresection and further surgery [1–7].

Muscular Reconstruction

Using the fundamental reconstructive principle of replacing like with like, it behooves the reconstructive surgeon to plan for the potential structures removed. The redundancy of lower extremity musculature does not always require resected musculature to be replaced to achieve adequate function, but when motor-unit defects are present following tumor resection, tendon transfers or functional muscle transfers can restore joint mobility. *En bloc* resection of the quadriceps muscles as a result of a soft tissue sarcoma in the anterior compartment may require functional muscle transfer to recover knee extension. The use of innervated contralateral vastus lateralis, gracilis, or hamstring muscle, or latissimus dorsi have all been described to achieve knee extension. Planning for this eventuality is imperative, as ambulation is the primary endpoint of limb salvage procedures [8, 9].

Arterial and Venous Reconstruction

Arterial and venous resection are often required when removing soft tissue sarcomas, requiring assistance from the vascular surgeon. Though venous ligation does not interfere with limb preservation, reconstruction can prevent long-term post-thrombotic syndrome and venous insufficiency. Venous revascularization remains controversial, however, because high occlusion rates are reported. Arterial resections, on the other hand, require reconstruction to avoid ischemia. Options for reconstruction include autografts (saphenous vein grafts), synthetic grafts, or allografts [10].

Nerve Reconstruction

Resection of nerves is frequently a consequence of limb salvage therapy. Every effort should be made to repair motor nerves, whereas smaller sensory nerves can be trimmed, infiltrated with lidocaine, and dunked into a muscle bed to avoid the formation of a neuroma. When nerve ends can be approximated in a tension-free manner, epineurial repair should be performed, using an end-to-end coaptation or end-to-side repair when the proximal nerve stump is unavailable. In the event of a nerve gap or tension during a primary repair, nerve grafting or tubulization should be performed. Autografts are the gold standard for bridging gaps, despite donor site morbidities. The sural nerve, medial antebrachial cutaneous nerve, lateral antebrachial cutaneous nerve, and superficial sensory branch of the radial nerve are all commonly used donors. Allografts or tubulization techniques are also viable options for repairing nerve injuries with gaps [11].

Dead Space Reconstruction, Prosthesis Coverage, and Cutaneous Reconstruction

The reconstructive surgeon is frequently called to fill dead space, cover implanted prostheses, or transfer tissue to achieve wound closure. Following resection of lesions, the surgeon frequently encounters dead space. Local muscle flaps are often viable options for medium-size defects of the lower extremity. Tensor fascia lata myocutaneous flaps, soleus flaps, gastrocnemius flaps, reverse sural flap, and medial plantar artery flap provide good solutions to achieve dead space control, prosthesis coverage, and local wound closure. Free autologous tissue transfer using anterolateral thigh flaps, radial forearm, gracilis, or the rectus abdominus can also reliably bring healthy, vascularized tissue into irradiated beds, cover prosthetics, or fill dead space.

Cutaneous reconstruction of the lower extremity depends on the location of the defect, its size, and the history of radiation to the wound. In the thigh, most skin defects can be closed if they are small enough. As the defects become larger, local flaps such as keystone and rhomboid flaps can be used for closure of the skin. In many instances, skin grafts can be placed onto muscle of the thigh if the bed is well vascularized. Besides local flaps, another option can be complex closure, with the placement of closed suction drains to eliminate the formation of seroma and hematoma.

Skin defects around the knee requiring soft-tissue reconstruction can be repaired with local muscle flaps such as the gastrocnemius muscle, with or without skin grafts. Mid-leg skin defects not able to be closed primarily can be closed with local muscle flaps such as the soleus and anterior tibialis muscle. Larger skin defects in the middle leg with exposure of bone and/or hardware will require free-tissue transfer if pedicled muscle flaps are not available. Skin defects in the lower third of the leg typically require free tissue transfer. This can take the shape of any fasciocutaneous flap tailored to the size of the skin defect. For example, these flaps can include the radial forearm flap, anterolateral thigh flap, deep inferior epigastric perforator flap, superficial circumflex iliac artery perforator flap, or any piece of skin with a named perforator or axillary blood vessel emanating from it. Skin defects of the ankle, heel, and foot can be reconstructed with free flaps of skin or muscle, but local flaps can suffice if defects are small enough. Cutaneous reconstruction of the lower extremity follows a thoughtful approach to close the wound in a tension-free manner, obliterate dead space, and cover exposed hardware or bone. In the setting of non-vascularized bone reconstruction for oncological defects, skin defects must be covered with well-vascularized tissue, either in a pedicle or as free tissue transfer. Location in the thigh versus the proximal, middle, or distal third of the leg dictates requirements for final reconstruction.

Postoperative Care

Postoperative weight-bearing status is typically determined by the orthopedic surgeon, especially when resection involves bony components. Extremity stabilizing devices are generally required, and their placement should be considered by the reconstructive surgeon. Time to healing must be considered in the patient's rehabilitation efforts. Radiation therapy may result in fibrosis and wound healing complications that require vigilant and continued care. Debulking procedures to address contour irregularities can be performed once treatment is complete.

Summary

Reconstruction of osteocutaneous defects requires detailed planning and collaboration with the oncologic surgeon. The repair of nerves, vascular structures, muscle function, and bony segments; coverage of prostheses; and filling of dead space are all components of patient-tailored limb-salvage procedures.

References

1. Rosenberg SA, Tepper J, Glatstein E, Costa J, Baker A, Brennan M, et al. The treatment of soft-tissue sarcomas of the extremities: prospective randomized evaluations of (1) limb-sparing surgery plus radiation therapy compared with amputation and (2) the role of adjuvant chemotherapy. Ann Surg. 1982;196:305–15.
2. Crago AM, Brennan MF. Principles in management of soft tissue sarcoma. Adv Surg. 2015;49:107–22.
3. Azadgoli B, Carre AL, Perrault DP, Wong AK. Complex reconstruction of the lower extremity following sarcoma resection: a literature review. Plast Aesthet Res. 2018;5:3. Available at: https://parjournal.net/article/view/2371. Accessed 4 Mar 2019.
4. Yang Y, Han L, He Z, Li X, Yang S, Yang J, et al. Advances in limb salvage treatment of osteosarcoma. J Bone Oncol. 2017;10:36–40.
5. Ogura K, Miyamoto S, Sakuraba M, Fujiwara T, Chuman H, Kawai A. Intercalary reconstruction after wide resection of malignant bone tumors of the lower extremity using a composite graft with a devitalized autograft and a vascularized fibula. Sarcoma. 2015;2015:861575. https://doi.org/10.1155/2015/861575.
6. Sewell MD, Hanna SA, McGrath A, Aston WJ, Blunn GW, Pollock RC, et al. Intercalary diaphyseal endoprosthetic reconstruction for malignant tibial bone tumours. J Bone Joint Surg Br. 2011;93:1111–7.
7. López JF, Hietanen KE, Kaartinen IS, Kääriäinen MT, Pakarinen TK, Laitinen M, Kuokkanen H. Primary flap reconstruction of tissue defects after sarcoma surgery enables curative treatment with acceptable functional results: a 7-year review. BMC Surg. 2015;15:71.

8. Walley KC, Taylor EM, Anderson M, Lozano-Calderon S, Iorio ML. Reconstruction of quadriceps function with composite free tissue transfers following sarcoma resection. J Surg Oncol. 2017;115:878–82.
9. Muramatsu K, Ihara K, Miyoshi T, Yoshida K, Hashimoto T, Taguchi T. Transfer of latissimus dorsi muscle for the functional reconstruction of quadriceps femoris muscle following oncological resection of sarcoma in the thigh. J Plast Reconstr Aesthet Surg. 2011;64:1068–74.
10. Nishinari K, Krutman M, Aguiar Junior S, Pignataro BS, Yazbek G, Zottele Bomfim GA, et al. Surgical outcomes of vascular reconstruction in soft tissue sarcomas of the lower extremities. J Vasc Surg. 2015;62:143–9.
11. Siemionow M, Brzezicki G. Current techniques and concepts in peripheral nerve repair. In: Geuna S, Pierluigi T, Battiston B, editors. Essays on peripheral nerve repair and regeneration. International review of neurobiology, vol. 87. United States: Academic; 2009. p. 141–72.

Chapter 6
Reconstruction of the Diabetic Limb

Hyunsuk Peter Suh and Joon Pio (Jp) Hong

Soft tissue necrosis and infection of the lower extremity are common end-stage events for the diabetic patient. Recent advances in microsurgical techniques have allowed surgeons to consider performing complex reconstructions in these patients. A carefully constructed preoperative assessment and plan are critical for success in this setting.

Scope of the Problem

Complications related to diabetic foot ulcers remain one of the most common reasons for diabetic patients' hospitalization. About one in four diabetic patients has a foot ulcer, and one out of five ulcers requires a major amputation [1]. Intractable diabetic foot ulcers can not only impair

H. P. Suh · J. P. (Jp) Hong (✉)
Department of Plastic and Reconstructive Surgery, Asan Medical Center, University of Ulsan College of Medicine, Seoul, South Korea
e-mail: joonphong@amc.seoul.kr

S. T. Hollenbeck et al. (eds.), *Handbook of Lower Extremity Reconstruction*, https://doi.org/10.1007/978-3-030-41035-3_6

Table 6.1 Purposes of flap surgery in diabetic limb reconstruction

Maximize length of limb
Near normal gait without prosthesis
Return to previous daily life
Minimize the mortality

physical, emotional, and social function but also impose substantial economic burdens for the patient and society [2]. Furthermore, the mortality rate for major amputations over 5 years can be as high as 80%. Successful surgical reconstruction and limb salvage using a microvascular free flap has been reported not only to preserve limb length and normal gait but also to significantly increase the 5-year survival rate [3, 4] (Table 6.1).

Although the recent increase in the success of limb salvage has improved patients' quality of life and rates of survival, the flap survival rate in diabetic foot reconstruction was reported to be 91.7%, much lower than the usual free flap success rate [3]. To minimize the failure rate of reconstructive surgery and help the patient to regain normal gait and go back to ordinary life, surgeons should thoroughly investigate the risk factors and underlying condition, including both the patient's general condition and local factors.

The Singularity of the Diabetic Foot

The spectrum of diabetic ulcer ranges from superficial ulceration to a critically ischemic limb or a severely infected wound with osteomyelitis. The reconstructive algorithm in Fig. 6.1 can guide the surgeon to make the proper choices for reconstruction.

The principal pathogenesis involving the diabetic ulcer will differ and may further increase the risk of flap surgery and morbidity during limb salvage procedures. Poor diabetes control, vasculopathy, renal failure, use of an immunosuppressive agent, the amount of soft tissue infection, the pres-

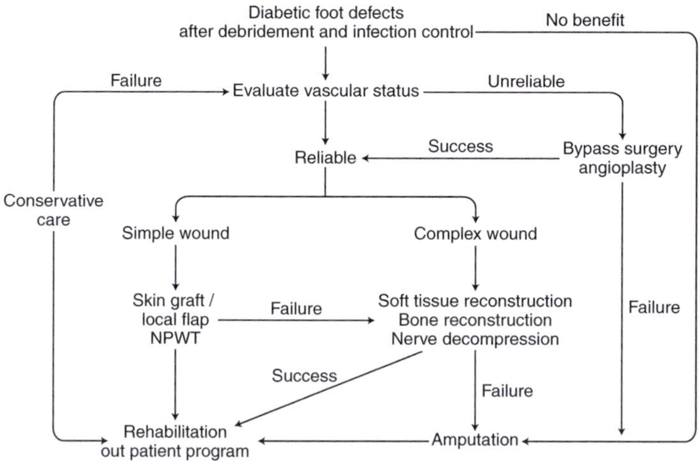

Figure 6.1 Algorithm for diabetic foot reconstruction. NPWT negative pressure wound therapy

ence of heart disease or osteomyelitis, and many other risk factors can contribute to the difficulties of flap surgery. Thus, the surgeon must evaluate the risks involved and work to correct them prior to surgery [5]. The two most prominent risk factors involved with flap success are vasculopathy and infection.

Diabetic Vasculopathy

Nearly 50% of patients with diabetic ulcer have shown some degree of vasculopathy, and 12% were found to have critical limb ischemia [6, 7]. In patients with vasculopathy, thorough vessel evaluation should be performed. If severe atherosclerosis is found in the target recipient vessel closest to the defect, the surgeon should dissect a distant peripheral vessel as a new recipient vessel and harvest a long pedicle flap, or should perform a bypass graft.

Preoperative Evaluation of Flow and Tissue Perfusion

CT angiography, conventional angiography, and color Doppler are the standard methods to evaluate the vascular status. With CT angiography, the surgeon can assess not only the peripheral vessel but also the calcification of major vessels, including superficial femoral artery, and even the condition of the donor vessel. In some cases with circumferential calcification, the lumen of the peripheral vessel cannot be seen, and the vasculopathy could be exacerbated. With conventional angiography, the obstruction can be checked and the volume of flow through the vessel also can be indirectly measured. A skilled interventionist can perform intraluminal angioplasty with minimal radioactive dye in patients with impaired renal function.

Management of Infection and Inflammation

Patients with diabeteshave immunopathies, with an abnormal immune response and an increased susceptibility to infection, which can quickly aggravate tissue necrosis. Inflammation itself also increases the pressure of the tissue, and when the increased pressure is higher than the capillary pressure, tissue necrosis occurs. In patients with sensory neuropathy, a foot ulcer can be neglected for a couple of days, and infection occurs, which can be aggravated rapidly along the fascia and soft tissue, causing severe infection and tissue necrosis.

Serial Surgical débridement with Tissue Culture

When patientsarrive at the hospital, timely, aggressive management can stop the progression of infection and preserve the maximal length of the limb, with the goal of limb salvage. Initial débridement should be performed within 12 hours of arrival, focusing on the removal of infected necrotic tissue and identifying the pocket and dead space under the skin. One should consider the angiosome concept when débriding the ischemic diabetic foot [8, 9]. Healthy, viable tissue should be achieved after removing the non-viable tissue. Pus or fluid covering the tissue should be washed out or removed by dry gauze. Additional débridement should be planned on the basis of the condition of the wound bed after the first débridement. If inflamed tissue remains, or the viability of the tissue is suspicious, a secondary surgery should be planned within the next 2 hours.

The Use of Antibiotics

Deep tissue culture is begun during the initial débridement, before starting empirical antibiotics. Empirical antibiotics generally are initially used for diabetic foot infections; the treatment is then changed to match bacterial culture results (Table 6.2). If the wound and infection do not change even

Table 6.2 Antibacterial therapy for infected diabetic foot ulcers

Severity of infection	**Antibacterial regimen**
Not limb-threatening (oral antibiotics)	Amoxicillin/clavulanic acid (500/125 mg) q8h Clindamycin 300 mg q6h Ciprofloxacin 500 mg q12h + clindamycin 300 mg q6h Dicloxacillin or flucloxacillin 500 mg q6h Levofloxacin 500 mg QD + clindamycin 300 mg q6h
Limb-threatening (parenteral)	Clindamycin 450–600 mg q6h + ciprofloxacin 400 mg q12h ± metronidazole 500 mg q8h Piperacillin/tazobactam 4.5 g q6h
Life-threatening (parenteral)	Piperacillin/tazobactam 4.5 g q6–8h + gentamicin 1.5 mg/kg q8h Vancomycin 1 g + gentamicin + metronidazole

after surgical débridement and antibiotics, a remnant pocket should be sought with additional débridement or MR imaging. Antibiotic resistance should considered, and the regimen changed to other antibiotics on the basis of systemic symptoms, wound condition, and blood tests.

The Timing of Flap Coverage After Vascular Intervention

Flap coverageshould be considered within 1 week after angioplasty or bypass surgery, as the rate of bypass failure cumulatively increases as the days pass. In a patient with severe ischemia who has successful revascularization, however, the reperfusion insult is higher during the subsequent 2 or 3 days than in a less ischemic limb or if revascularization is not successful. If it is suspected before revascularization that reperfusion insult and inflammatory reaction are likely, flap coverage surgery should be scheduled after an interval of at least 2–3 days.

The Timing of Flap Coverage After Infection Control

Wound preparation should be done correctly before the flap coverage. If active inflammation remains under the flap, it is not possible to drain the inflamed discharge or minimize the bacterial count with methods such as negative pressure dressing or surgical débridement. At a minimum, there should be no skin redness caused by soft tissue inflammation, and no purulent discharge from the dead space. The use of NPWT (negative pressure wound therapy) can help one identify whether the wound is ready for the next stage of reconstruction by demonstrating good granulation.

Soft Tissue Reconstruction

Once the wound preparation is done and reasonable tissue perfusion is achieved, soft tissue flap coverage is considered for patients with an extensive and complex wound. Bone exposure is a common reason for reconstruction. Local flaps can be considered for reconstruction of small wounds that are not responsive to conservative or advanced care. To ensure flap survival, one must evaluate the circulation of the foot, however, as the use of a local flap may devastate the distal flow if the vascularity is scarce in the foot. For complex wounds, free flaps may offer the best chance for salvage. The most valuable indication is for reconstruction of an amputation stump or heel reconstruction; proximal amputation is inevitable for many of these cases without the flap surgery (Figs. 6.2, 6.3, and 6.4).

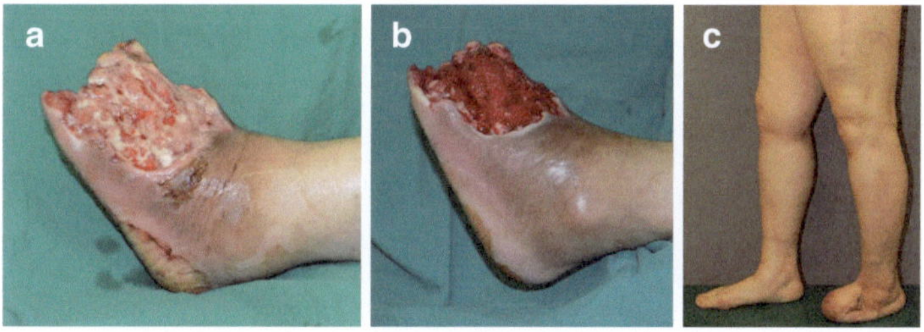

FIGURE 6.2 A 49-year-old diabetic woman referred to for limb salvage. (**a**) After toe amputation, necrotic tissue was covering the wound bed. (**b**) After wound débridement and angioplasty, the wound bed is free of necrotic tissue and covered with granulation tissue. (**c**) After removal of necrotic bone, a perforator flap was used to cover the trans-metatarsal amputation stump, and the flap was free of re-ulceration after 3 years

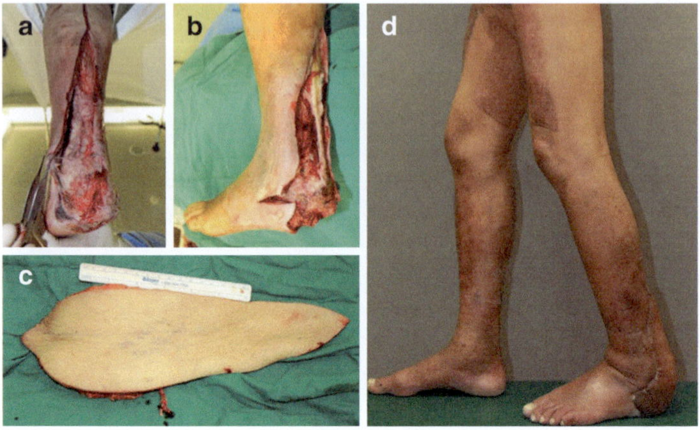

FIGURE 6.3 A 51-year-old man had a severe infection on his left leg, with a high fever. A local hospital recommended emergency below-knee amputation. He was transferred for limb salvage. (**a**) Emergency débridement was performed, and all the dead space was exposed. (**b**) After several wound débridements in a week, the wound was free of necrotic tissue and inflammation. Calcaneal bone was exposed. (**c**) An anterolateral thigh (ALT) flap was elevated, with a fascial strip for reconstruction of the Achilles tendon defect due to severe necrosis. (**d**) The left lower leg was salvaged, and normal gait was possible with tolerable ankle motion

Recipient Vessel Selection

Finding a good recipient vessel for proper perfusion of the flap is both the most challenging thing and the most important factor in successful flap reconstruction. A pulsatile signal or acoustic wave from handheld Doppler does not guarantee a good recipient vessel for anastomosis. The sensitivity of handheld Doppler is very high; it can trace a vessel less than 0.2–0.3 mm in diameter, which cannot meet the physiologic demand for flap survival. The surgeon should look for the vessel based on anatomical knowledge and a preoperative radiologic study, along with intraoperative Doppler tracing.

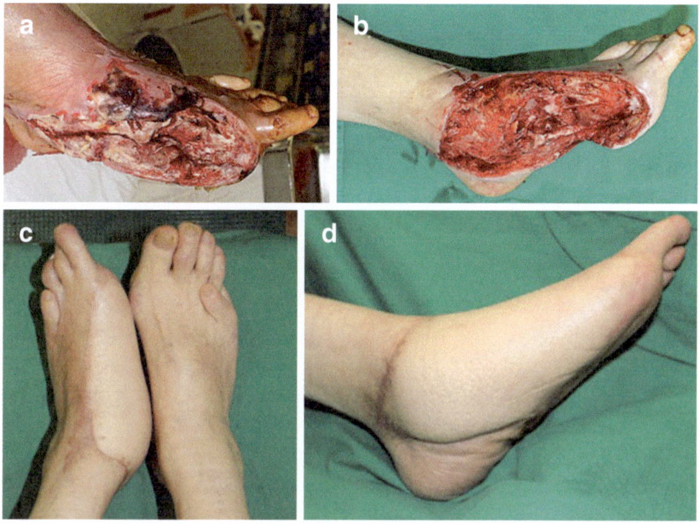

FIGURE 6.4 A 67-year-old woman had a small wound on the first toe of her left foot after clipping the toenail; it became infected within a week. She had a systemic infection, and laboratory findings showed an elevated inflammatory reaction. (**a**) She was referred to the clinic because of aggravation of the wound even after first toe ray amputation. (**b**) Serial débridement was performed, with negative pressure wound dressing. Bone and joint space were exposed. (**c**, **d**) The defect was covered with ALT perforator flap, and she was free from recurrence after 3 years and 6 months

If the vessel has adequate flow for the anastomosis, the pulsation of the vessel can be seen under the loupe magnification, but there may be no visible pulsation if there is severe calcification in the long segment. In this situation, handheld Doppler helps to evaluate the flow within the calcified vessel. Small branches (0.5–1 mm) from the dorsalis pedis or digital artery can be used for end-to-end anastomosis in forefoot reconstruction, which can be called *supermicrosurgery* [4, 10]. A small branch from the pedal artery is usually free of atherosclerosis and calcification in most cases when the flow is maintained in severely calcified pedal arteries. If there is a peripheral artery, medial plantar artery, lateral plantar artery, or dorsalis pedis artery within or near the defect, it can be used with an end-to-side method or flow-through method.

Flap Selection

The flap should be well vascularized after surgery, so it can stand up against the remaining inflammation under the flap and in the wound bed. The flap should also tolerate shear stress from shoes and pressure during weight-bearing. Muscle flaps with skin grafts can be an acceptable option, but we prefer perforator flaps for most soft tissue defects in diabetic limb salvage, including plantar surface reconstruction, because of their thin and durable character. Again, the most important step remains proper wound bed preparation before the flap coverage. The perforator flap has many advantages for limb salvage, and it also minimizes the donor site complications and morbidity. The anterolateral thigh (ALT) perforator flap (Figs. 6.3, 6.4) or superficial circumflex iliac artery perforator (SCIP) (Fig. 6.5) is preferred for most cases because it can be thin, pliable, and durable [11, 12]. For the small to moderate-size defect, the SCIP flap is the flap of choice.

Microanastomosis and Vessel Insetting

In our experience, one of the reasonsfor flap failure in diabetic reconstruction is arterial occlusion, which is more likely than in other flap surgeries. Because of calcification and phosphate deposition in the medial and intimal wall, the intimal wall is already injured before the anastomosis, and the result may be higher rates of postoperative thrombus formation after the microanastomosis and vascular procedures.

If the artery used for end-to-side anastomosis is severely calcified, we try to find a 5-mm length of the spared lesion for

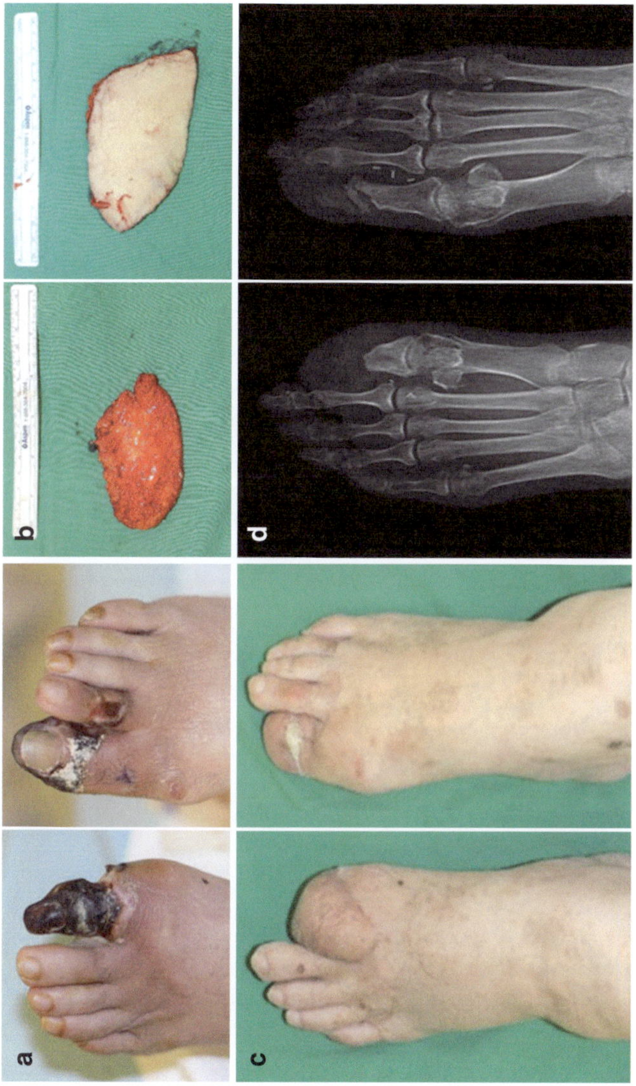

FIGURE 6.5 **(a)** A 61-year-old woman had dry necrosis of both big toes caused by a burn. **(b)** Bilateral superficial circumflex iliac perforator (SCIP) flaps were elevated. The flaps were connected to the dorsal digital artery just proximal to the defect on both sides. **(c)** The flap was free from ulceration after 2 years and 8 months. **(d)** The bone was free from the osteomyelitis. During ambulation, the patient had normal plantar pressure to the forefoot and minimal additional pressure to the tip

anastomosis. If a spared segment cannot be seen or if calcification remains on the vessel media, Dafilon® 9–0 monofilament suture (B. Braun Medical; Bethlehem, PA, USA), which has a strong 5-mm needle, can be used. After the successful anastomosis, the vessel should be placed with extra care. If the recipient vessel and end-to-side–anastomosed donor pedicle are calcified, there is a higher chance of compression and kinking than in a non-calcified vessel, which may lead to vessel occlusion.

Selection of Patients

To minimize morbidity during the salvage procedure and flap surgery, cases should be selected on the basis of the patient's underlying condition and the skill of the surgeon. Low flow volume and low pressure of the recipient vessel are common in diabetic foot reconstruction, and vessel calcifications are typical in a diabetic wound with vasculopathy. To preserve the flow to the rest of the foot, and to prevent iatrogenic ischemia, use of a small branch from a peripheral vessel or end-to-side anastomosis to the peripheral vessel is an essential surgical procedure. If the surgeon is not familiar with this method, the chance of flap failure will be increased, aggravating the ulcer and infection, and perhaps even leading to proximal amputation.

Summary

In the authors' reports [3, 4], the algorithm of managing the diabetic ulcer with a free flap showed flap survival of more than 91% and a limb salvage rate of 84.9%. The 5-year survival rate was 86.8%. Serial débridement, infection control, vascular intervention, and proper use of initial empirical antibiotics can be combined with a multidisciplinary approach and the effort of the medical staff.

References

1. Singh N, Armstrong DG, Lipsky BA. Preventing foot ulcers in patients with diabetes. JAMA. 2005;293:217–28.
2. Apelqvist J. Wound healing in diabetes. Outcome and costs. Clin Podiatr Med Surg. 1998;15:21–39.
3. Oh TS, Lee HS, Hong JP. Diabetic foot reconstruction using free flaps increases 5-year-survival rate. J Plast Reconstr Aesthet Surg. 2013;66:243–50.
4. Suh HS, Oh TS, Hong JP. Innovations in diabetic foot reconstruction using supermicrosurgery. Diabetes Metab Res Rev. 2016;32(Suppl 1):275–80.
5. Endara M, Masden D, Goldstein J, Gondek S, Steinberg J, Attinger C. The role of chronic and perioperative glucose management in high-risk surgical closures: a case for tighter glycemic control. Plast Reconstr Surg. 2013;132:996–1004.
6. Jude EB, Oyibo SO, Chalmers N, Boulton AJ. Peripheral arterial disease in diabetic and nondiabetic patients: a comparison of severity and outcome. Diabetes Care. 2001;24:1433–7.
7. Suh HP, Kim Y, Suh Y, Hong J. Multidetector computed tomography (CT) analysis of 168 cases in diabetic patients with total superficial femoral artery occlusion: is it safe to use an anterolateral thigh flap without CT angiography in diabetic patients? J Reconstr Microsurg. 2018;34:65–70.
8. Attinger CE, Bulan EJ. Débridement. The key initial first step in wound healing. Foot Ankle Clin. 2001;6:627–60.
9. Attinger CE, Evans KK, Bulan E, Blume P, Cooper P. Angiosomes of the foot and ankle and clinical implications for limb salvage: reconstruction, incisions, and revascularization. Plast Reconstr Surg. 2006;117(7 Suppl):261S–93S.
10. Suh HS, Oh TS, Lee HS, Lee SH, Cho YP, Park JR, et al. A new approach for reconstruction of diabetic foot wounds using the angiosome and supermicrosurgery concept. Plast Reconstr Surg. 2016;138:702e–9e.
11. Hong JP. Reconstruction of the diabetic foot using the anterolateral thigh perforator flap. Plast Reconstr Surg. 2006;117:1599–608.
12. Goh TL, Park SW, Cho JY, Choi JW, Hong JP. The search for the ideal thin skin flap: superficial circumflex iliac artery perforator flap – a review of 210 cases. Plast Reconstr Surg. 2015;135:592–601.

Chapter 7
Technological Advances to Simplify Lower Extremity Reconstruction

Dennis P. Orgill and Mahendra Daya

Introduction

The introduction of early free-tissue transfer to treat open fractures of the lower extremity was a great advance in reconstructive surgery and has dramatically reduced amputation rates, but these procedures require a high degree of technical skill and have the large disadvantage of failure rates of 1–10%. Failures can be catastrophic when the entire flap becomes necrotic and must be removed. Free flaps also necessarily place a scar on another area of the body and can substantially reduce function when a large muscle is taken. These flaps are often bulky and require revision. A recent revolution of new technologies can assist the reconstructive surgeon who is treating both traumatic and non-traumatic wounds.

D. P. Orgill (✉)
Division of Plastic Surgery, Brigham & Women's Hospital, Harvard Medical School, Boston, MA, USA
e-mail: dorgill@partners.org

M. Daya
Department of Plastic and Reconstructive Surgery, Inkosi Albert Luthuli Central Hospital, Mayville, South Africa

S. T. Hollenbeck et al. (eds.), *Handbook of Lower Extremity Reconstruction*, https://doi.org/10.1007/978-3-030-41035-3_7

Negative Pressure Wound Therapy (NPWT) Devices

These devices most often consist of a foam covered by a semi-occlusive dressing that is connected to a suction source (also referred to as vacuum-assisted closure; Fig. 7.1). They have become a standard dressing to be placed on traumatic wounds following initial débridement. The dressings can isolate the wound from external contamination and induce the formation of granulation tissue. They reduce excess edema and keep the wound moist. The powerful ability to induce granulation tissues can cover areas of bone, cartilage, and tendon. Adding irrigation with saline allows for a nice effect in contaminated wounds.

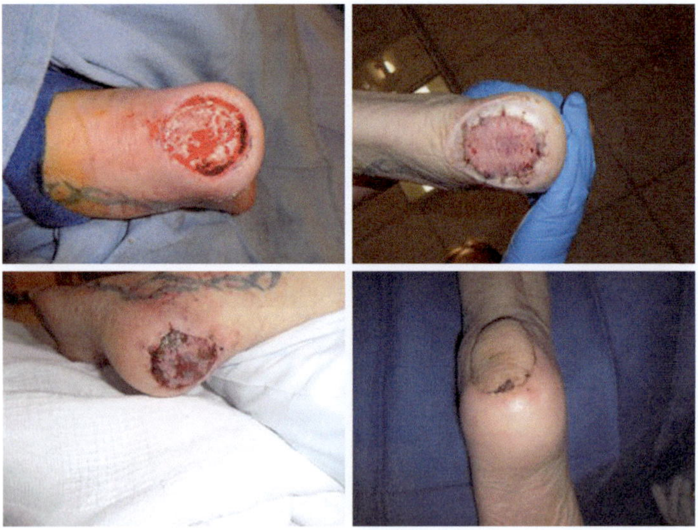

Figure 7.1 Infected Achilles tendon treated by drainage and V.A.C. VERAFLO™ device (Acelity, San Antonio, TX) for 5 days, followed by a skin graft

Tape Dermatogenesis and Tissue Expansion

Tissue expansion in the lower extremity can be an effective method to generate additional skin, but needs to be used with substantial caution. Simple taping of skin around wounds allows a similar effect with reduced surgeries (Fig. 7.2). This technique is gaining application throughout the world. Initially pioneered to resurface large scars of the scalp, it is currently being used in many other areas of skin deficiency.

Bioengineered Skin

Two products on the market in the United States, Apligraf® and Dermagraft® (Organogenesis, Canton, MA) are bioengineered skin substitutes that have been effectively used on chronic wounds (Fig. 7.3).

Placenta-Derived Constructs

A number of placenta-derived constructs are on the market today with clinical trials demonstrating efficacy (Fig. 7.4). These include sheets derived from the amnion, chorion, umbilical cord, or combinations of materials. Some products are cryopreserved and others are dehydrated.

Dermal Scaffolds

A number of dermal scaffolds have been developed that are either semi-synthetic or derived from human or animal tissues. A porous collagen-glycosaminoglycan scaffold with a silicone membrane has been quite useful in treating areas with small areas of exposed tendon or bone (Fig. 7.5). These constructs are often used in conjunction with a NPWT device.

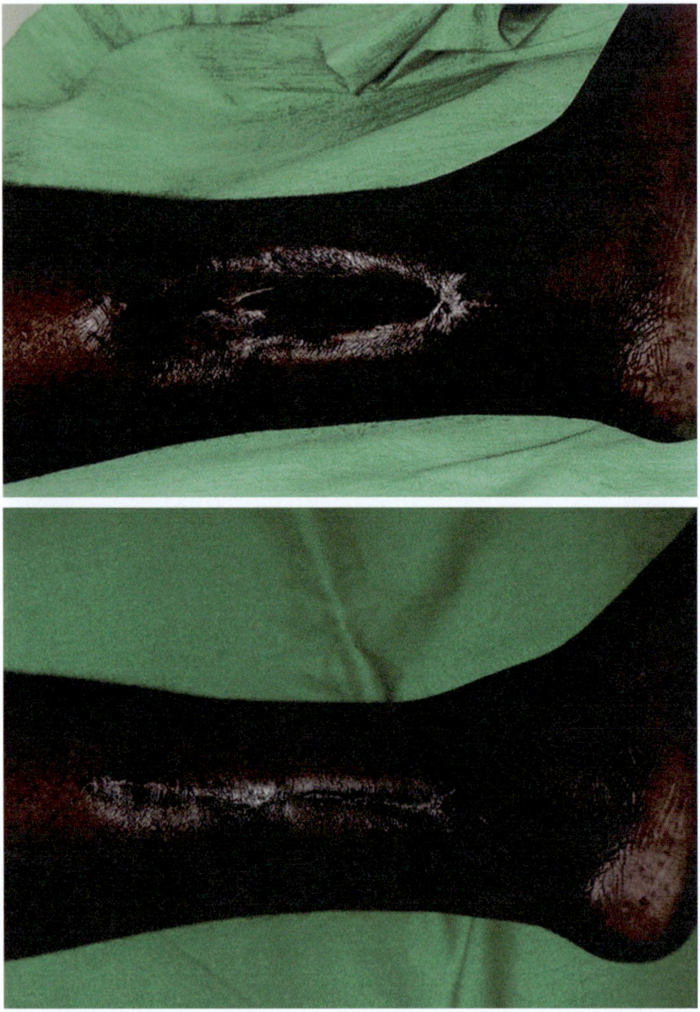

Figure 7.2 (*Top*) A contour deformity on the lower third of the medial aspect of the leg. (*Bottom*) A good correction of the deformity is noted at 3 months. (*From* Daya M, Nair V. Traction-assisted dermatogenesis by serial intermittent skin tape application. *Plast Reconstr Surg*. 2008;122:1047–54; with permission)

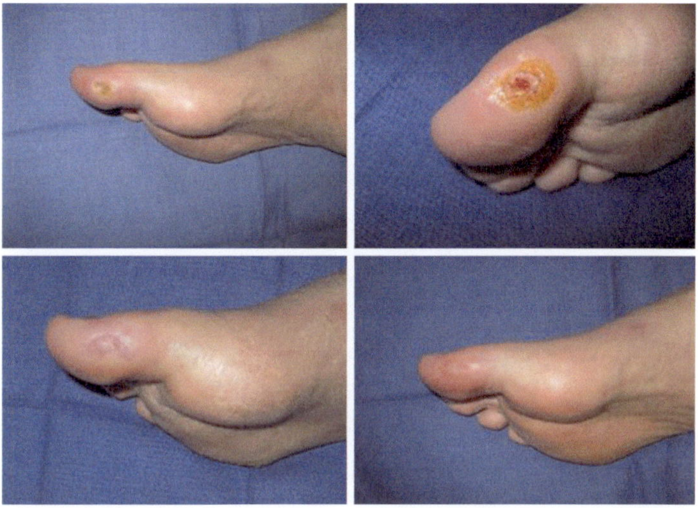

FIGURE 7.3 Superficial toe ulcer treated with bioengineered bi-layered skin substitute. *Top left*, Initial ulcer; *Top right*, 1 week after initial treatment; *Bottom left*, 4 weeks; *Bottom right*, At 3 months

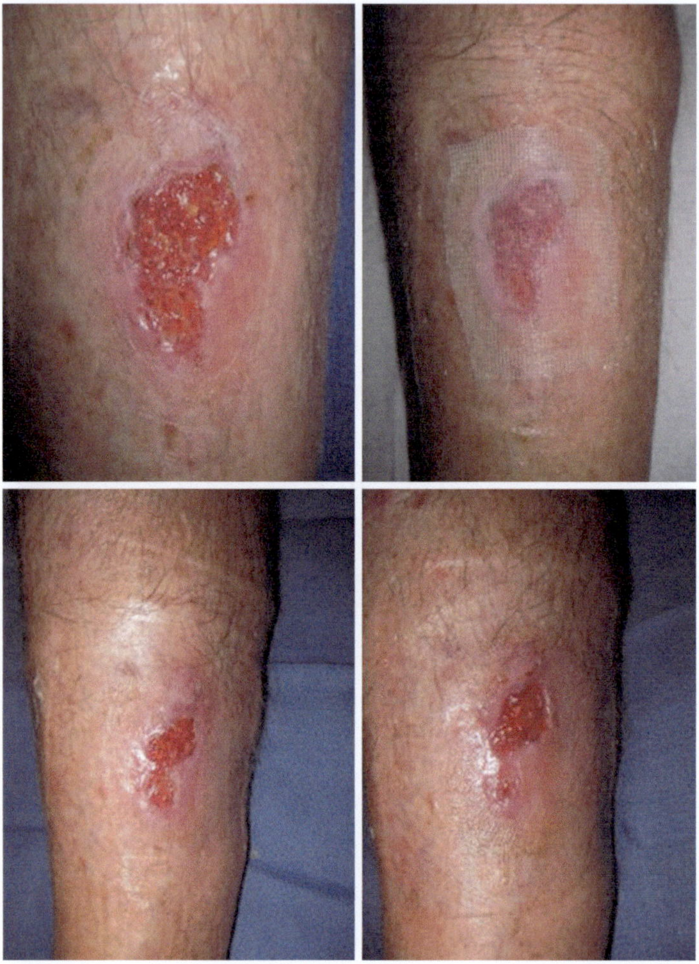

FIGURE 7.4 Superficial ulcer treated with cryopreserved placental membrane. Chronic non-healing ulceration of the anterior tibial area treated with weekly applications of a cryopreserved amniotic allograft. *Top left*, Initial wound after debridement; *Top right*, 1 week after first application; *Bottom left*, 2 weeks after first application; *Bottom right*, 3 weeks after initial application

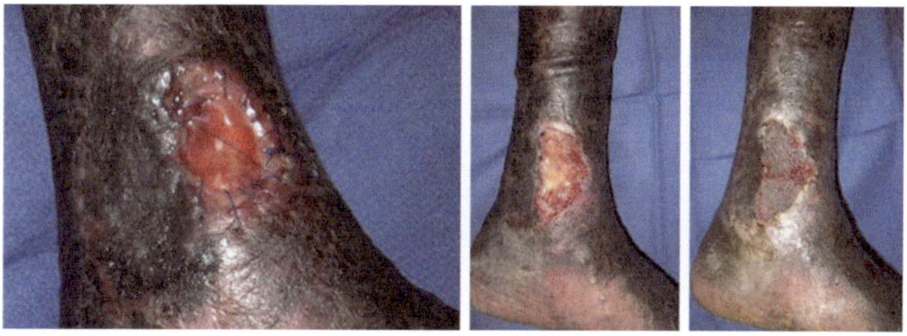

Figure 7.5 Sarcoid ulcer treatment with dermal matrix (Integra®; Integra LifeSciences, Plainsboro, NJ). (*Left*) Wound after treatment with Integra®, immediate aspect. (*Center*) Four-week aspect after implanting Integra®. (*Right*) Split-thickness skin graft 1 week post-operatively. (*From* Climov M, Bayer LR, Moscoso AV, Matsumine H, Orgill DP. The role of dermal matrices in treating inflammatory and diabetic wounds. *Plast Reconstr Surg*. 2016;138(3 Suppl):148S–57S; with permission)

Summary

Technological advances have dramatically altered practice patterns in lower extremity wounds. These include NPWT, bioengineered skin substitutes, and dermal scaffolds. In parallel, advances in flap reconstruction, including perforator flaps, now give surgeons many local and regional options for wound closure. These techniques are valuable not only for the complex wound following trauma but also for certain chronic wounds. Further clinical trials and registry studies will be important to better guide clinicians in the future.

Chapter 8
Flap Principles Applied to Lower Extremity Reconstruction

Bryan J. Pyfer, Rebecca Vernon, and Scott T. Hollenbeck

Lower extremity reconstruction is unique in that there is high variability in tissue types and demands throughout the leg. Many soft tissue defects will involve concomitant bony injury, so an orthoplastic approach is required. Once it is determined that flap reconstruction is required, there are three main considerations:

- timing
- type of flap
- technical execution of the procedure to produce a reliable outcome

Timing for flap coverage remains one of the most debated topics in this field. In general, the sooner the better. The pri-

B. J. Pyfer
Division of Plastic Surgery, Duke University Hospital, Durham, NC, USA

R. Vernon
Division of Plastic, Maxillofacial, and Oral Surgery, Department of Surgery, Duke University School of Medicine, Durham, NC, USA

S. T. Hollenbeck (✉)
Division of Plastic and Reconstructive Surgery, Duke Medical Center, Durham, NC, USA
e-mail: scott.hollenbeck@duke.edu

S. T. Hollenbeck et al. (eds.), *Handbook of Lower Extremity Reconstruction*, https://doi.org/10.1007/978-3-030-41035-3_8

mary mechanism and extent of the defect will drive the decision making for flap selection. In smaller defects or those associated with minimal energy, local flaps and other non-flap approaches may be reasonable and effective, but for significant defects associated with high-energy injuries or prior field radiation, free tissue transfer will be needed. In the setting of trauma, when limb salvage has been deemed appropriate and débridement has been completed, a plan for flap reconstruction is needed. This chapter is designed to guide the surgeon in that process.

Muscle vs. Fasciocutaneous Flaps

Ideally when reconstructing a wound, the replacement of "like with like" provides the best functional and structural outcome, but in instances of trauma or cancer, particular tissue types may have unique advantages. Historically, muscle flaps were regarded as superior to fasciocutaneous flaps, but current literature supports similar rates of limb salvage and functional recovery for both muscle and fasciocutaneous flaps [1]. This finding has led to a significant paradigm shift over the past two decades towards fasciocutaneous flaps. Still, a wide variety of flaps may be useful for lower extremity reconstruction and at times may be required because of extraneous factors such as other comorbidities (Fig. 8.1).

Muscle flaps have the theoretical advantage of contouring to the irregularities of a defect. Flaps like the latissimus dorsi can be spread out over large areas and remain relatively thin. Its high metabolic activity and degree of vascularization make muscle relatively resistant to infection [2]. This quality may be important when there are exposed fracture sites or hardware in the wound, or if the wound is at high risk for infection. The donor sites of muscle-only flaps can almost always be closed primarily and tend to have acceptable aesthetic outcomes. Indeed, muscle flaps often become thinner over time owing to muscle atrophy, although in ambulatory patients, one must carefully weigh the impact of sacrificing

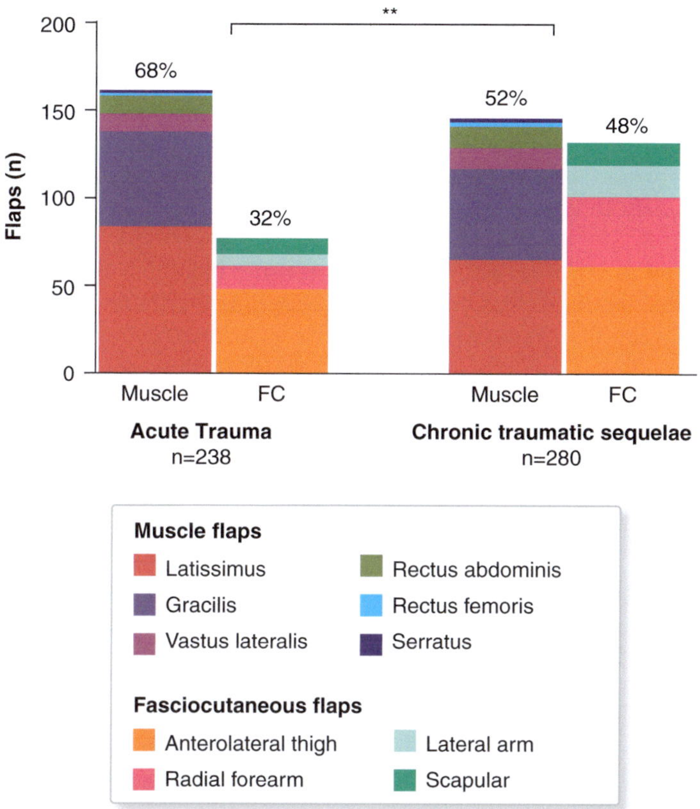

FIGURE 8.1 Distribution of muscle and fasciocutaneous lower extremity free flaps performed at two high-volume centers over a 17-year period. (*From* Cho et al. [1], with permission)

functional muscle for soft tissue coverage. Additionally, muscle can sometimes be too bulky and have poor aesthetic outcomes. The need for split-thickness skin grafts often leads to an irregular appearance and inflexible construct that may limit motion, especially if the flap extends over a joint.

Conversely, fasciocutaneous and perforator flaps have the benefit of being thin and pliable. Their numerous potential donor sites allow for a variety of reconstructive options, but there is a higher degree of variability in the anatomy of lipocutaneous and fasciocutaneous perforators. This variability can be planned for preoperatively with vascular imaging, or intraoperatively with pencil Doppler ultrasound. Fasciocutaneous flaps preserve muscle function and have few, if any, functional donor deficits, leading to reduced postoperative recovery time and shorter hospitalization stays. They may be less resistant to infection than muscle flaps, however, and may be prone to isolated areas of fat necrosis. Also, aesthetic results at the donor site may be poor if they can't be closed primarily and require skin grafting. Skin flaps do have one specific advantage in that they do not stick down to the deep spaces with as much scar as muscle flaps. This is important if subsequent flap elevation and orthopedic procedures (such as bone grafting) are anticipated.

Flap Timing

Flap timing continues to be highly debated in the literature. Priorities in reconstructive efforts should center first on vascular sufficiency, debridement of nonviable tissue, stability of underlying structures (i.e. bony fixation), and infection control. Early research by Godina from the 1980s showed that in acute trauma patients with Gustilo grade IIIb/c fractures, limb salvage rates were higher when coverage was obtained within 72 hours after injury [3]. More recent studies, however, show that similar outcomes can be achieved even if flaps are performed outside of this traditional window [4, 5]. Modern advances in wound care technology, including negative pressure wound therapy (NPWT), allow for stable temporary coverage of open wounds. This permits reconstruction to be postponed until conditions are more optimal. In soft tissue defects from cancer, some debate exists as to whether flap surgery should take place before or after chemotherapy or radiation therapy. As of now, there is no clearly established time-frame for reconstruction, but generally speaking, modern reconstructive practice suggests that the sooner the reconstruction takes place, the better the outcome for the patient.

Local vs. Free Flaps

The location and type of defect, combined with patient-specific systemic factors, will largely determine whether a local or free flap is a more suitable reconstructive option. Traditionally, local flaps have been preferred for defects of the thigh and the proximal two thirds of the leg, where there is substantial muscular redundancy. For instance, for a proximal thigh defect, one could sacrifice the vastus lateralis, tensor fascia lata, gracilis, or rectus femoris muscles (to name a few), with little functional deficit. As one moves more distally in the leg, local options become more limited. Prior to the popularization of pedicled perforator flaps, defects of the distal third of the leg almost always necessitated a free flap. The increased use of perforator flaps has allowed for more local reconstructive options for all zones of the lower extremity.

Small wounds or minimal-energy wounds with healthy surrounding tissue often can be treated with local flaps (Fig. 8.2). High-energy, irradiated, or chronic wounds are more likely to have a large zone of injury, and the transfer of well-vascularized tissue from a distant source may be necessary. These conditions may preclude local reconstruction.

Finally, patient-specific systemic factors should always guide treatment. Young or advanced age is not a contraindication *per se*, but one must consider the patient's ability to withstand the prolonged anesthesia required for free tissue transfer. Smoking impairs wound healing, and patients should be encouraged to stop smoking 2 to 4 weeks prior to elective free flap surgery, if possible [6]. Patient reliability should be assessed, as free flaps require a greater willingness to comply with a strict postoperative rehabilitation regimen.

Hypercoagulable disorders are a relative contraindication to free flaps. Elevated preoperative platelet count has been shown to predict risk of thrombosis in acute lower extremity trauma, with higher platelet counts correlating with higher risk for microvascular complications (Fig. 8.3) [7, 8]. Preoperative platelet counts may therefore aid in patient risk stratification and surgical decision making in this setting. It is

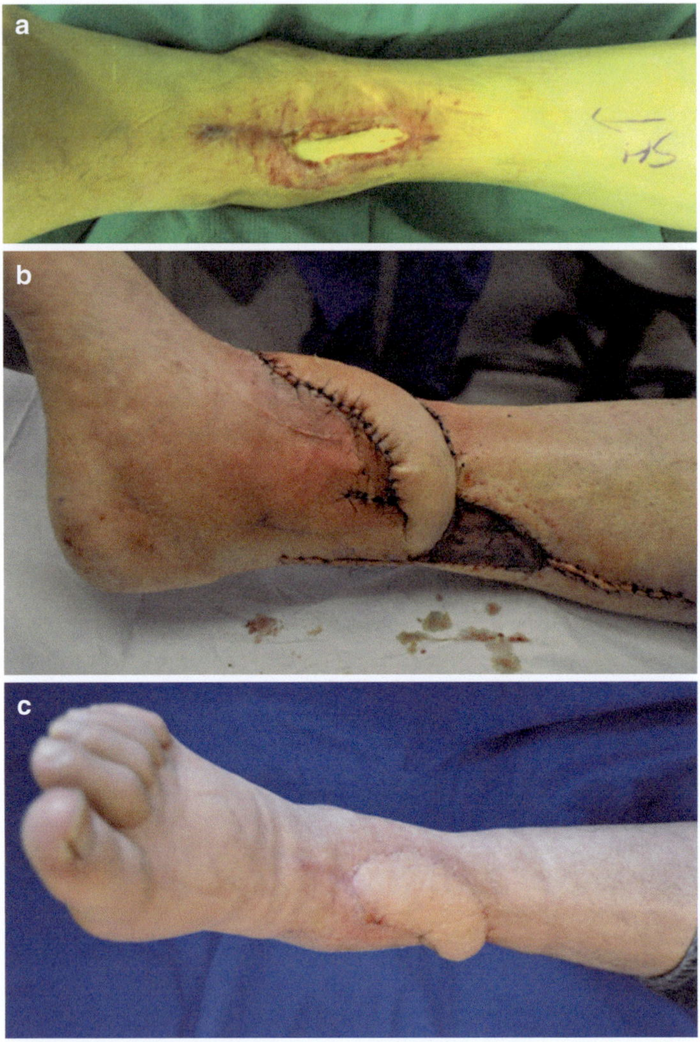

FIGURE 8.2 Posterior tibial artery perforator peninsula flap. (**a**) This 60-year-old man had wound breakdown and an exposed tibialis anterior tendon 6 weeks after a total ankle replacement. (**b**) The defect has been closed with a posterior tibial artery perforator peninsula flap with split-thickness skin graft to the donor defect. (**c**) The final result is shown 6 weeks post-op

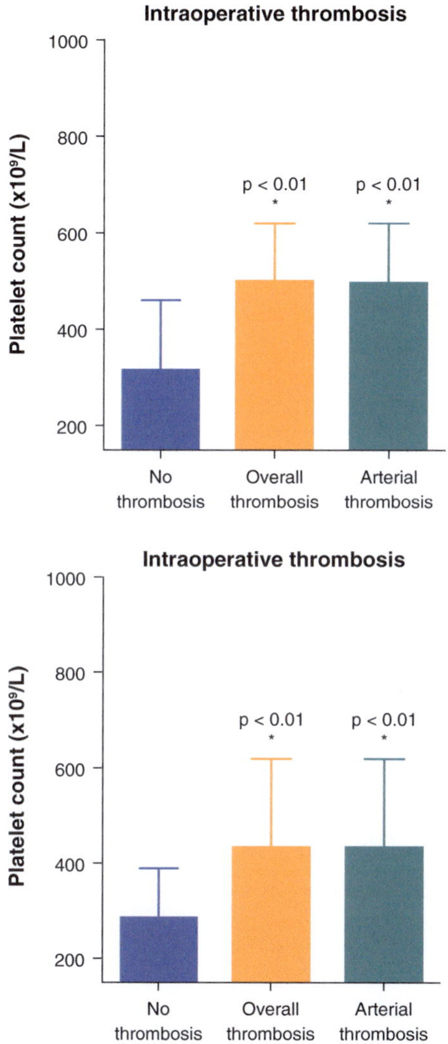

FIGURE 8.3 Intraoperative thrombotic complications, according to preoperative platelet counts. (*Top*) Acute trauma patients (n = 215). (*Bottom*) Patients who did not sustain acute trauma (n = 350). Data are expressed as mean +/– standard deviation. Statistical comparisons were performed relative to the routine intraoperative course with no thrombosis. Intraoperative venous thrombosis is not shown because of low incidence (n = 1). (*From* Cho et al. [7], with permission)

also suggested that selective anticoagulation may improve microsurgical outcomes in high-risk patients with thrombophilia or other hypercoagulable conditions.

Overall Free Flap Approach

After a patient is deemed a suitable candidate for free flap reconstruction, careful analysis of the flap's recipient and donor sites must take place. The cause, size, and location of the defect will generally guide surgical planning. Flap components should ideally match those missing from the defect. In high-energy trauma wounds and wounds in irradiated beds, typically much more tissue is required than one might suspect initially. Nonviable, avascular, or damaged tissue must be excised prior to definitively selecting a flap, in order to accurately understand the true size of the defect. Consideration must also be given as to whether radiation to or through the flap is expected in the future, as one should plan to have enough tissue bulk to withstand inevitable radiation changes to the flap. In defects from cancer, cancer margins should be negative and final before free flap reconstruction takes place.

Appropriate selection of flap recipient vessels is critical to flap survival, so arterial and venous sufficiency of the recipient site should always be investigated prior to surgery. This is especially true in the elderly (who suffer a high incidence of atherosclerotic disease) or with concomitant orthopedic trauma, where vessels may have been injured. Preoperative CT angiography (CTA) is not generally required but often is helpful in patients with manifestations of peripheral vascular disease or following trauma. An abnormal (or highly limited) ankle-brachial index or pulse exam mandates preoperative CTA or MR angiography (MRA) [6].

If peripheral vascular disease or vessel trauma in or around a defect would otherwise preclude the use of certain flaps with shorter vascular pedicles, a vein graft can be used to extend the reach of the pedicle. Vein grafts are also useful to allow the anastomosis to reach outside the zone of injury (Fig. 8.4). A vein graft harvest site should be planned preop-

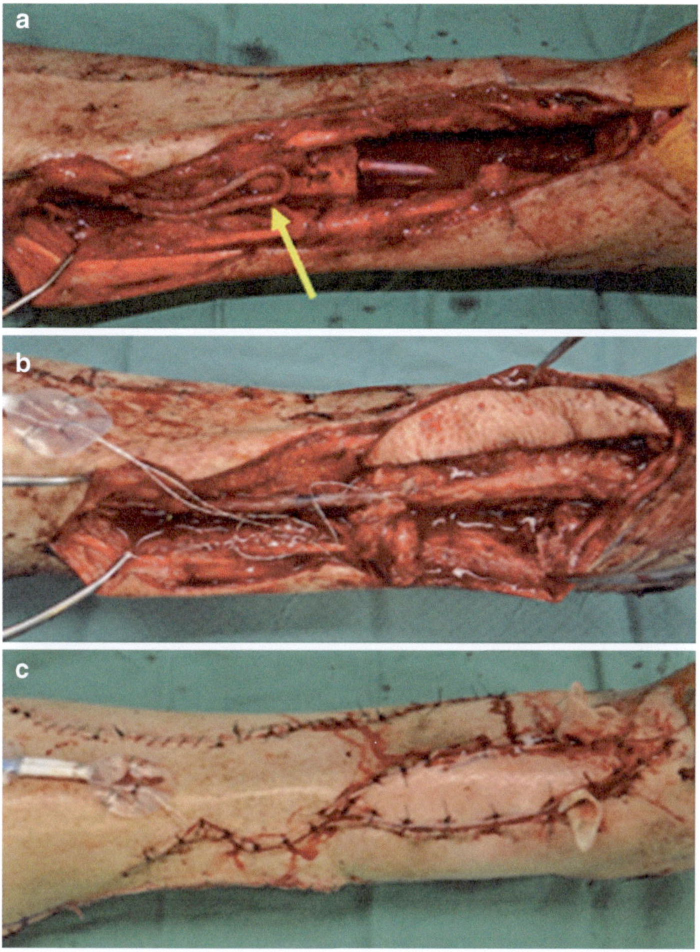

Figure 8.4 Ipsilateral free osteocutaneous fibula flap with vein graft for ankle fusion. (**a**) The distal leg following multiple failed surgeries for ankle fusion. The distal tibia has been removed. An intramedullary nail is present. A vein graft has been performed, in the form of an AV loop (*arrow*) to the proximal anterior tibial vessels. (**b**) The pedicle of the osteocutaneous fibula flap has been coapted to the AV loop. (**c**) The defect has been closed with the fibula flap skin paddle facing the anterior leg

eratively, even if it is not definitely needed, and the site should be surgically prepared and draped at the beginning of the case.

Donor vessels should be a similar size match, and a thorough medical and surgical history and physical examination should be performed to ensure that no previous surgeries or conditions could have compromised the pedicle of the proposed flap.

Technical Considerations for Free Flaps

As for any free flap, vessel size-matching and anastomotic technique can impact flap selection and surgical approach. Significant size mismatches between donor and recipient vessels have been shown to decrease laminar flow, increase turbulence and stasis, and ultimately increase the risk of thrombosis. Size discrepancy can be overcome by techniques like spatulation, wedge resection from the larger vessel, interposition vein grafting, or end-to-side anastomosis.

The decision between end-to-end and end-to-side anastomosis has been well studied in the literature, and there are no clear data to show that either has better outcomes [9]. The choice of anastomotic technique should be guided by patient and clinical factors, such as the extent of tissue damage and the quality and accessibility of recipient vessels. End-to-side anastomoses are generally preferred in the setting of compromised vascular status, as in patients with peripheral vascular disease or diabetes, but an end-to-end anastomosis is typically easier to perform and may be done proximal to a vessel injury to avoid concern about leg devascularization. Generally speaking, leg devascularization is extremely rare in the setting of flap reconstruction unless there is single-vessel run-off to the foot [9].

A common pitfall for lower extremity free flap reconstruction is insufficient skin, resulting in a tight closure. This may not manifest until post-op day 1 or 2, when the venous outflow becomes compromised secondary to external pressure. To avoid this complication, the flap should be designed with adequate tissue to cover the pedicle and allow for a tension-free closure and the challenge of subsequent edema.

Postoperative Care

For any number of reasons, soft tissue reconstruction may be needed prior to bony fixation of orthopedic fractures, which necessitates the postoperative use of an external fixator. The placement of an external fixator after pedicled or free flap reconstruction should always be approached with extreme caution, and only as a joint effort between the orthopedist and the plastic surgeon who placed the flap. External fixators can also be used as a "kick stand" to hold the leg off the bed during recovery. This is especially important for flaps that are on the posterior foot or leg.

To allow for permanent flap integration while avoiding flap congestion, and to aid patient rehabilitation, intensive postoperative lower extremity flap protocols must be instituted and strictly followed by patients (Table 8.1). Most surgeons agree that some period of bed rest with lower extremity elevation is important in the earliest postoperative period, with gradual transition to progressive dangling and eventual ambulation. To improve contour and overall aesthetic (and sometimes functional) outcomes, lipocutaneous or fasciocutaneous flaps can be thinned either surgically or via liposuction. General timing for revision procedures is around 6 months after the initial flap surgery.

Table 8.1 Protocol for postoperative care of lower extremity free flaps at Duke University Division of Plastic and Reconstructive Surgery

Post op time	Diet	Activity	Movement of affected joints	Anticoagulation	Elevation & dangling
Day 0	NPO	Bedrest		Enoxaparin 40 mg daily. ASA 81 mg daily while inpatient & up to 1 month post-op	Leg elevated 3 pillows ("toes to nose")
Day 1	Clear		ROM of uninvolved joints		
Day 2	Regular diet				
Day 3		Out of bed to chair with PT: transfers to chair, bedside commode, wheelchair			Leg may dangle for transfers only. No weight bearing.

Day 5	Convert OR splint to orthoplast splint. Keep ankle in neutral with no pressure on flap.			
Day 7		ROM of joints in close proximity to affected joint		
Day 14		ROM of joints crossed by flap		End of strict leg elevation. Dangle 5 mins TID, increase by 5 mins daily.
1 month	Dependent training & ACE wrap		End anticoagulation	
1.5 months	Toe touch (pending orthopedic recommendation)			
2–3 months	Ambulate (pending orthopedic recommendation)			

References

1. Cho EH, Shammas RL, Carney MJ, Weissler JM, Bauder AR, Glener AD, et al. Muscle versus fasciocutaneous free flaps in lower extremity traumatic reconstruction: a multicenter outcomes analysis. Plast Reconstr Surg. 2018;141:191–9.
2. Kang MJ, Chung CH, Chang YJ, Chang YJ. Reconstruction of the lower extremity using free flaps. Arch Plast Surg. 2013;40:575–83.
3. Godina M. Early microsurgical reconstruction of complex trauma of the extremities. Plast Reconstr Surg. 1986;78:285–92.
4. Hill JB, Vogel JE, Sexton KW, Guillamondegui OD, Corral GAD, Shack RB. Re-evaluating the paradigm of early free flap coverage in lower extremity trauma. Microsurgery. 2013;33:9–13.
5. Karanas YL, Nigriny J, Chang J. The timing of microsurgical reconstruction in lower extremity trauma. Microsurgery. 2008;28:632–4.
6. Hollenbeck ST, Toranto JD, Taylor BJ, Ho TQ, Zenn MR, Erdmann D, Levin LS. Perineal and lower extremity reconstruction. Plast Reconstr Surg. 2011;128:551e–63e.
7. Cho EH, Bauder AR, Centkowski S, Shammas RL, Mundy L, Kovach SJ, et al. Preoperative platelet count predicts lower extremity free flap thrombosis: a multi-institutional experience. Plast Reconstr Surg. 2017;139:220–30.
8. DeFazio MV, Economides JM, Anghel EL, Tefera EA, Evans KK. Lower extremity free tissue transfer in the setting of thrombophilia: analysis of perioperative anticoagulation protocols and predictors of flap failure. J Reconstr Microsurg. 2018; https://doi.org/10.1055/s-0038-1675145. [Epub ahead of print].
9. Cho EH, Garcia RM, Blau J, Levinson H, Erdmann D, Levin LS, Hollenbeck ST. Microvascular anastomoses using end-to-end versus end-to-side technique in lower extremity free tissue transfer. J Reconstr Microsurg. 2016;32:114–20.

Chapter 9
Local Skin Flaps for Lower Extremity Wounds

Dennis P. Orgill, Andrew Atia, and Scott T. Hollenbeck

In the absence of extensive local trauma, edema, or radiation injury, local flaps may be a reasonable option for lower extremity reconstruction. When the defect is large and deep, a muscle flap may be required to obliterate the dead space, but when the defect is limited in its size and complexity, a local fasciocutaneous flap may suffice. These flaps can be elevated and positioned using a number of techniques described in this chapter.

D. P. Orgill
Division of Plastic Surgery, Brigham & Women's Hospital, Harvard Medical School, Boston, MA, USA

A. Atia · S. T. Hollenbeck (✉)
Division of Plastic and Reconstructive Surgery, Duke University Medical Center, Durham, NC, USA
e-mail: scott.hollenbeck@duke.edu

S. T. Hollenbeck et al. (eds.), *Handbook of Lower Extremity Reconstruction*, https://doi.org/10.1007/978-3-030-41035-3_9

Perfusion of the Skin

Skin is nourished by blood vessels that perforate the fascia or traverse muscle, arborize throughout the adipose layer, and then connect the subdermal and dermal plexus of the skin. These perforating vessels primarily nourish a specific area of skin referred to as an *angiosome*; they can be mapped out [1]. Because the skin has a relatively low metabolic demand, rather small perforators can supply a surprisingly large area of skin. The skin also has redundancy in its blood supply, making it generally possible for all the skin of a specific and adjacent angiosome to survive based on a single perforator. Our understanding of perforator flaps has largely replaced previous classification schemes that are geometrically based; all skin flaps are based to a certain extent on a perforator that supplies that region of skin.

Principles of Skin Flaps

Skin flaps have their own blood supply [2]. There must be adequate arterial inflow, perfusion, and venous outflow to avoid ischemia and necrosis. Early flaps were based on muscles and their proximal blood supply. The redundant and rich blood supply in muscles provides robust soft tissue coverage but has the disadvantage of sacrificing a functioning unit that provides mobility. Later, fasciocutaneous flaps were designed on the basis of a good independent blood supply to the fascia. Skin flaps have been used for years, with many theories advanced to predict how large of a flap will survive. We now realize that specific perforators directly perfuse the skin, allowing for great innovation in flap design. Once the perforator flap is dissected back to its source, it creates a large arc of rotation to transpose the flap to the desired location (Fig. 9.1). Current techniques allow further dissection of these vessels—including through muscles to large feeding vessels (pedicle)—to increase the arc or rotation.

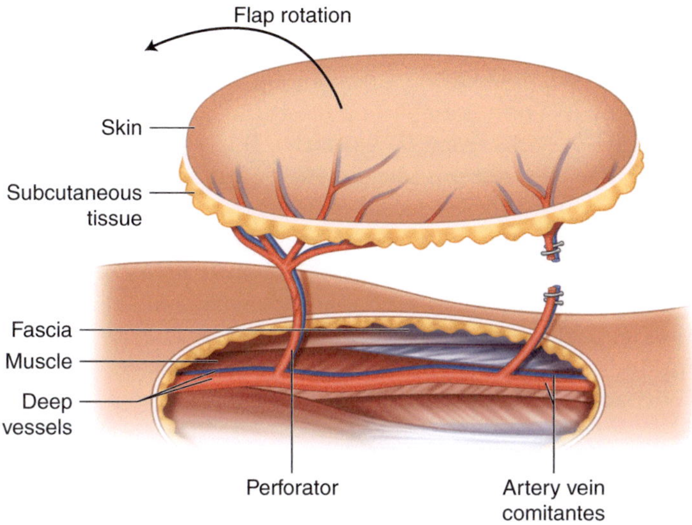

FIGURE 9.1 Schematic diagram of a local skin flap. Skin is vascularized from perforators through fascia and muscle that arborize through the subcutaneous tissue and skin and connect with an adjacent angiosome [3]. Dissection back to the perforator allows for a greater arc of rotation

Delay Principles: Skin and Vascular

The skin has the remarkable ability to generate new blood vessels over time, a process called *neovascularization*. The pathways for neovascularization are based on hypoxia [4]. One pathway involves hypoxia-inducible factor 1α that stimulates vascular endothelial growth factor (VEGF) production, resulting in new blood vessel formation [5]. This process starts a few days after surgery and peaks 2–3 weeks after surgery. The principle of vascular delay, whereby blood supply to a flap is disrupted in order to increase alternate blood supply to the tissue, has been used for nearly 500 years by the reconstructive surgeon [6]. Similarly, skin delay may be performed when a large area of skin is required for transfer by incising a limited proportion of the borders of an adjacent skin territory to allow neighboring choke vessels to mature. Local tissue blood supply can be enhanced by completing a flap delay procedure from 3 days to about 2 weeks prior to definitive flap surgery. For flaps where the vascular supply may be tenuous, doing a delay procedure prior to flap transfer can greatly enhance success. This principle has commonly been utilized in the lower extremity. For example, prior to reconstruction using the reverse sural flap (Fig. 9.2), the flap is partially raised and then sutured back *in situ* before definitive transfer several days or weeks later. Though delay procedures do have the drawback of delaying definitive coverage, they may be helpful in certain circumstances.

Perforator Flaps

There are a wide range of designs possible for flaps based on individual perforators. Perforator flaps allow the surgeon to design a flap specific to the defect, based on a nearby perforator. Each of the many perforators in the lower extremity has the capacity for the design of a flap, thus allowing a wide arrange of local options. Many of these lower extremity perforator flaps have been extensively studied, with multiple publications demonstrating the precise anatomy of the source perforators [7, 8]. These studies do show a variability in the anatomic location of most perforators. From a practical design standpoint, most surgeons will use a hand-held Doppler probe to identify the location of the perforator. They will then use the relative strength of the Doppler signal and exact location to make a more precise flap design. Once the perforator is found, the dissection is continued more proximal until sufficient length is established on the pedicle for rotation. A flap that will be rotated 180 degrees (a propeller flap) should have extra pedicle length to prevent twisting and vascular occlusion (Fig. 9.3).

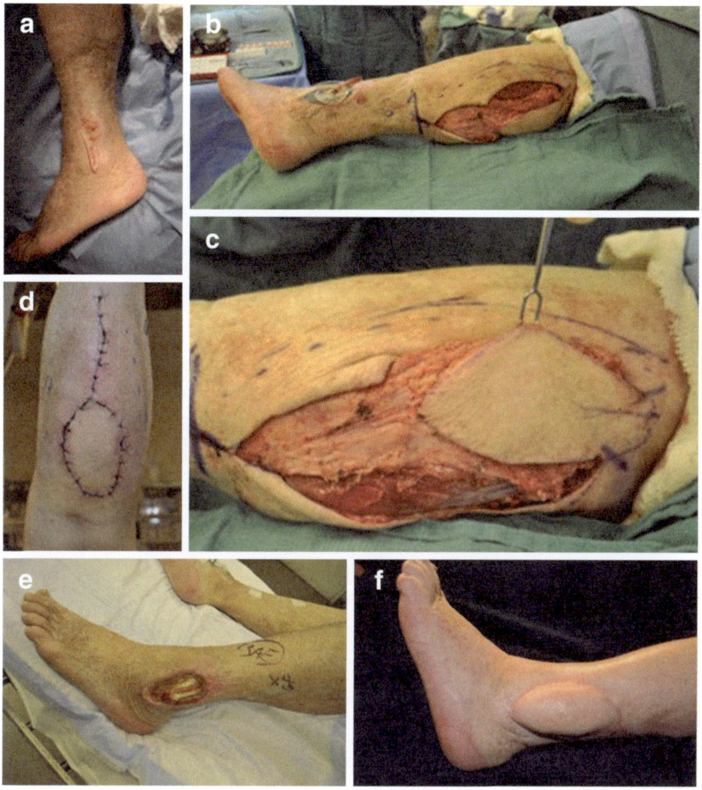

FIGURE 9.2 Reverse sural flap with skin and vascular delay. (**a**) A chronic wound of the lateral malleolus overlying hardware. (**b**) A delayed reverse sural flap is chosen for reconstruction. The sural flap is elevated and is supplied by the adipofascial pedicle from the distal extremity. (**c**) A proximal skin bridge is maintained at the time of surgery. (**d**) The skin bridge is incised at a later date in the office setting and re-inset. (**e**) A photo of the wound after débridement and negative pressure therapy. The flap is then completely re-elevated and used to reconstruct the defect. (**f**) The final reconstruction. (*Photos courtesy of* Scott T. Hollenbeck, MD)

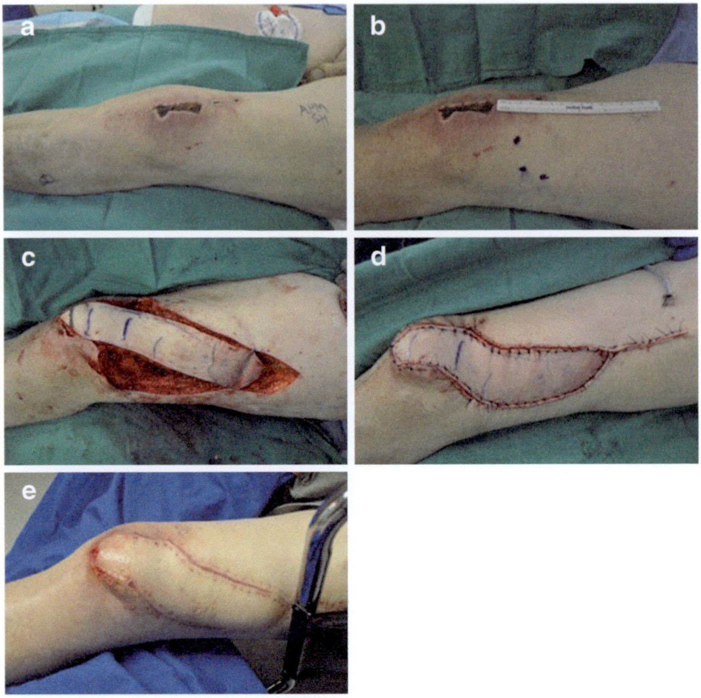

FIGURE 9.3 Propeller flap for knee coverage. (**a**) A chronic wound of the knee. (**b**, **c**) A propeller flap is designed around a central pedicle. The fasciocutaneous flap is then elevated and rotated into the defect. (**d**) The flap is then inset, and the donor site is closed primarily. (**e**) The final reconstruction after suture removal. (*Photos courtesy of* Scott T. Hollenbeck, MD)

Reverse Flaps

Understanding the vascular supply of various regions of the body is critical in the design of flaps. A reverse flap is an axial pattern flap that is based off of distal vessels. In these flaps, the proximal vascular supply is transected, and the flap is perfused from perforators that are based distally, which allows rotation of the flap to cover distal defects. Several lower extremity reverse flaps have been described in the literature, which serve as additional options for the reconstructive surgeon. Commonly used reverse flaps include the reverse sural flap, reverse anterolateral thigh flap, and the reverse first dorsal metatarsal artery flap (Fig. 9.4). For large reverse flow flaps that require significant rotation, the delay principles previously mentioned may be used to optimize survivability of the flap [9].

Geometric Design of Flaps

Advances in technology, including negative pressure wound therapy, scaffold technologies, and amniotic constructs, have allowed for temporizing measures for wound closure, which can shrink the size of the defect [10]. For many lower extremity injuries, the area of "required coverage" is substantially smaller than the entire original defect, making it possible to use local flaps to cover many defects [11]. A simple transposition flap to cover the exposed bone, with a skin graft covering the donor area, can be a simple method to restore skin coverage (Fig. 9.5a), but avoiding a skin graft has several advantages. Therefore a number of geometric designs have been proposed to close both the defect and the donor site created by moving the flap. The most common methods used have been described as V-Y advancement flaps (Fig. 9.5b) and Keystone flaps [12] (Fig. 9.5c).

The thigh has a robust blood supply with many perforating vessels located throughout the region. Often, plastic surgeons are faced with soft tissue defects around the knee, and perforating vessels on the genicular system or off the distal end of the descending branch of the lateral circumflex femoral (DBLCF) vessels can provide many options for knee coverage. Proximally based flaps based on the DBLCF can have a large arc of rotation and can cover substantial areas in the abdomen and pelvis. The posterior thigh also has several large perforators just below the gluteal crease that can be used for the treatment of ischial pressure injuries [13].

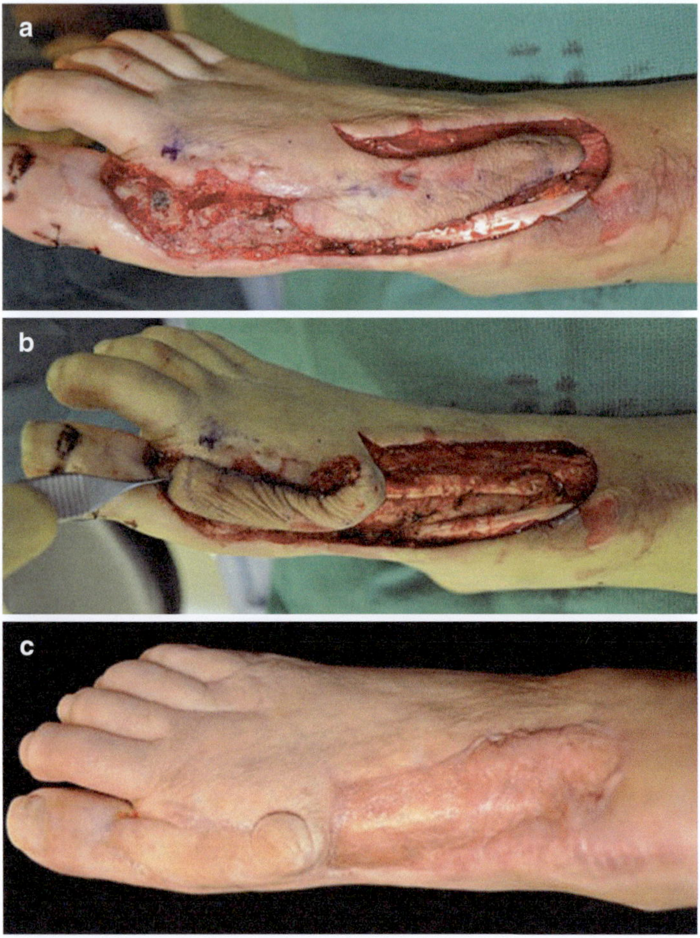

FIGURE 9.4 (**a**) Full-thickness skin loss to the dorsal surface of the foot with exposed extensor tendon and bone. For the foot, the dorsal metatarsal artery perforator flap can be used in a reverse fashion to cover toe lesions. (**b**) The flap is raised and rotated to cover the distal defect. A skin graft is then used to reconstruct the donor site. (**c**) The final reconstruction is shown 10 weeks after surgery. (*Photos courtesy of* Scott T. Hollenbeck, MD)

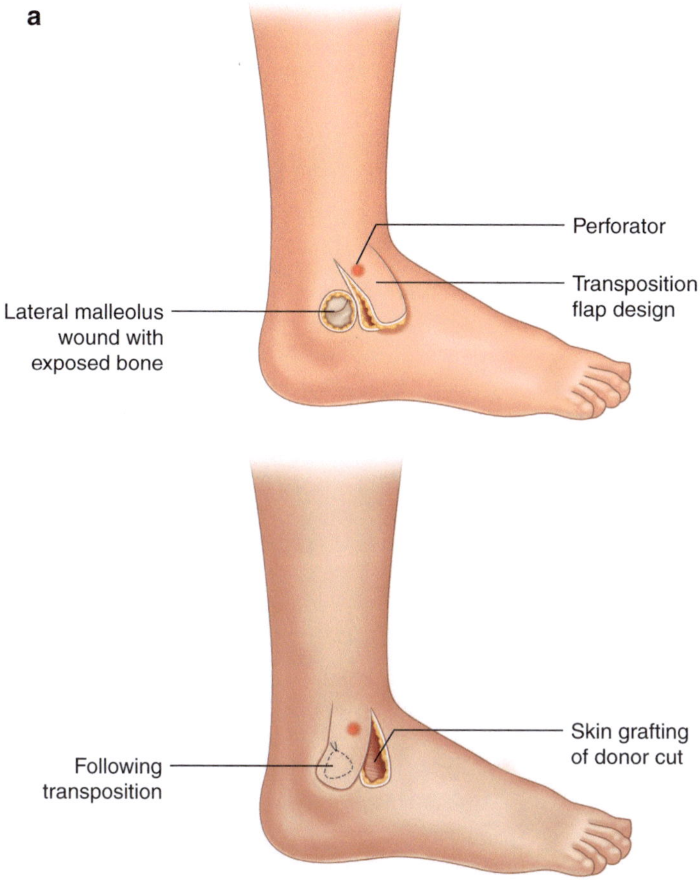

FIGURE 9.5 (**a**) The figure shows a wound of the lateral malleolus with exposed bone. A transposition flap is designed based off of a local perforator. The tissue is then elevated and rotated to cover the defect. A skin graft is then used to reconstruct the donor site. (**b**) Reconstruction of a wound using a V-Y advancement flap. A perforator is identified. A V-Y fasciocutaneous flap is dissected and advanced into the adjacent defect. The donor site is closed primarily. (**c**) Reconstruction of a wound using a Keystone flap. This flap is a multi-perforator flap that can be customized with incisions through skin only, or incisions through the deep fascia to allow minimal tension on the wound closure. As shown, a Keystone flap is dissected and advanced into the adjacent defect. The donor site is closed primarily

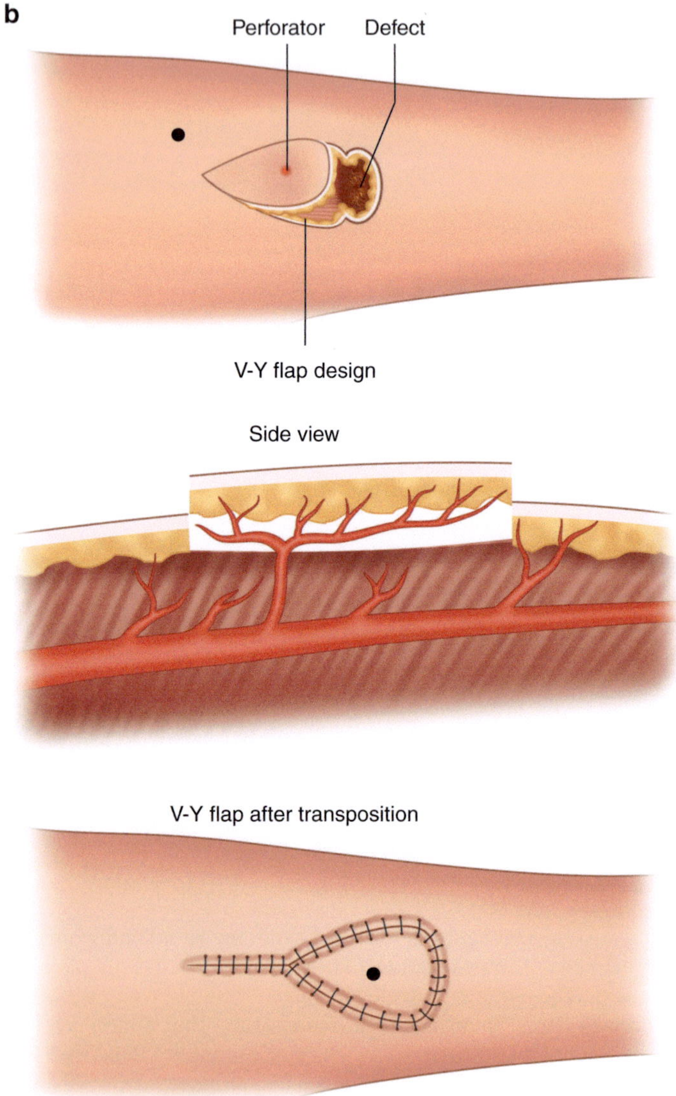

FIGURE 9.5 (continued)

c

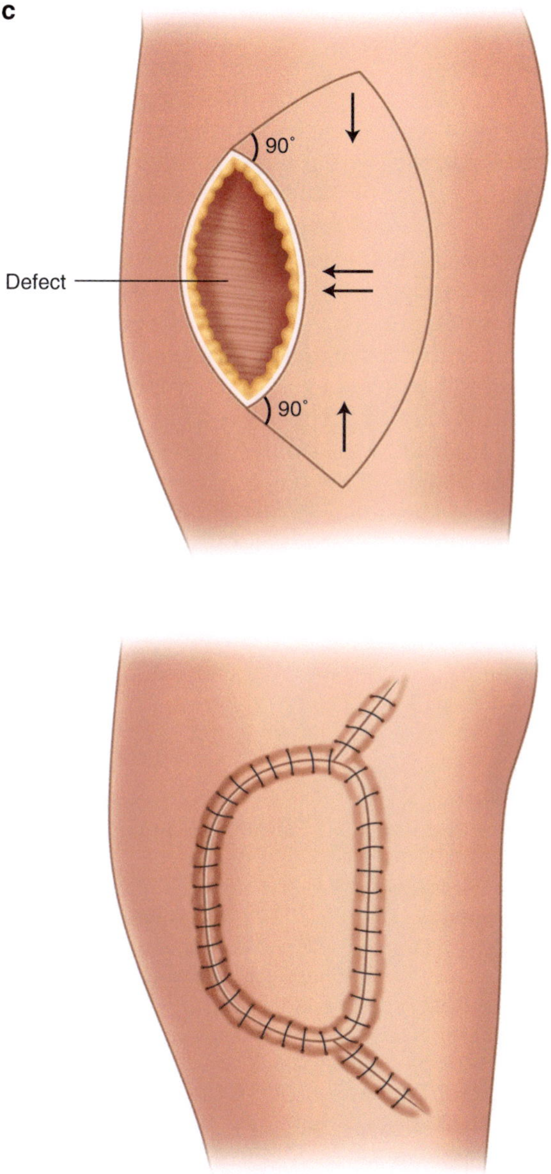

FIGURE 9.5 (continued)

Summary

Skin of the lower extremity is supplied by a number of large perforators that connect to well-described vascular structures. The precise location of these perforators has substantial variation between patients, but generally follows the basic angiosome principles. Identification of the perforators with a hand-held Doppler device or preoperative imaging with confirmation during the dissection can give the reconstructive surgeon a number of options when dealing with difficult problems of the lower extremity. As these perforating vessels are small, care must be taken during dissection to avoid injury, and during inset to avoid excessive tension or twisting of the pedicle. If the flap needs to be rotated 180 degrees, twisting can be minimized by distributing this rotation over a longer length of the pedicle. If the flap is congested, returning the flap to its original location and subsequently performing the rotation at a later date can be helpful. Additionally, the principles of vascular delay can be used to make marginally reliable flaps more robust, so that they can be used to perform a successful reconstruction.

References

1. Taylor GI, Palmer JH. The vascular territories (angiosomes) of the body: experimental study and clinical applications. Br J Plast Surg. 1987;40:113–41.
2. Koshima I, Soeda S. Inferior epigastric artery skin flaps without rectus abdominis muscle. Br J Plast Surg. 1989;42:645–8.
3. Saint-Cyr M, Wong C, Schaverien M, Mojallal A, Rohrich RJ. The perforasome theory: vascular anatomy and clinical implications. Plast Reconstr Surg. 2009;124:1529–44.
4. Fong GH. Regulation of angiogenesis by oxygen sensing mechanisms. J Mol Med (Berl). 2009;87:549–60.
5. Ferrara N, Gerber HP, LeCouter J. The biology of VEGF and its receptors. Nat Med. 2003;9:669–76.
6. Ghali S, Butler PE, Tepper OM, Gurtner GC. Vascular delay revisited. Plast Reconstr Surg. 2007;119:1735–44.

7. Almeida MF, da Costa PR, Okawa RY. Reverse-flow island sural flap. Plast Reconstr Surg. 2002;109:583–91.
8. Yu P. Characteristics of the anterolateral thigh flap in a Western population and its application in head and neck reconstruction. Head Neck. 2004;26:759–69.
9. Kneser U, Bach AD, Polykandriotis E, Kopp J, Horch RE. Delayed reverse sural flap for staged reconstruction of the foot and lower leg. Plast Reconstr Surg. 2005;116:1910–7.
10. Moues CM, van den Bemd GJ, Heule F, Hovius SE. Comparing conventional gauze therapy to vacuum-assisted closure wound therapy: a prospective randomised trial. J Plast Reconstr Aesthet Surg. 2007;60:672–81.
11. Capobianco CM, Zgonis T. An overview of negative pressure wound therapy for the lower extremity. Clin Podiatr Med Surg. 2009;26:619–31.
12. Mohan AT, Rammos CK, Akhavan AA, Martinez J, Wu PS, Moran SL, et al. Evolving concepts of keystone perforator island flaps (KPIF): principles of perforator anatomy, design modifications, and extended clinical applications. Plast Reconstr Surg. 2016;137:1909–20.
13. Lin H, Hou C, Chen A, Xu Z. Long-term outcome of using posterior-thigh fasciocutaneous flaps for the treatment of ischial pressure sores. J Reconstr Microsurg. 2010;26:355–8.

Chapter 10
Principles of Local Muscle Flaps for Lower Extremity Wounds

Andrew L. Peredo, Matthew L. Iorio, and David W. Mathes

Lower extremity wounds can be secondary to a variety of sources, including trauma, oncologic resection, neuropathy, or vascular disease, so they can require a variety of techniques for successful reconstruction. This chapter discusses some of the local muscle flaps generally utilized for lower extremity wounds.

Principles of Muscle Flaps

Muscle flaps are advantageous because they can obliterate dead space with well-vascularized tissue [1]. Muscle flaps are defined based on the origin of their vascular supply. The size, location, and number of vascular pedicles often influences flap design in order to ensure the survival of the muscle. The vascular pedicles of the muscle are defined as dominant

A. L. Peredo · D. W. Mathes (✉)
Department of Surgery, Division of Plastic and Reconstructive Surgery, University of Colorado, Anschutz Medical Campus, Aurora, CO, USA
e-mail: david.mathes@cuanschuz.edu

M. L. Iorio
Division of Plastic Surgery, University of Colorado Hospital, Aurora, CO, USA

S. T. Hollenbeck et al. (eds.), *Handbook of Lower Extremity Reconstruction*, https://doi.org/10.1007/978-3-030-41035-3_10

(when there are multiple pedicles present) or major (when more than one pedicle is dominant). Minor pedicles are the nondominant pedicles. Secondary pedicles are segmental minor pedicles that can support the flap despite ligation of a dominant major pedicle. The most accepted classification system of the circulatory patterns of muscle flaps is the Mathes and Nahai Classification [2].

The lower leg below the knee can be divided into thirds, with the proximal and middle thirds efficiently closed with local muscle flaps (Fig. 10.1). The distal third, however,

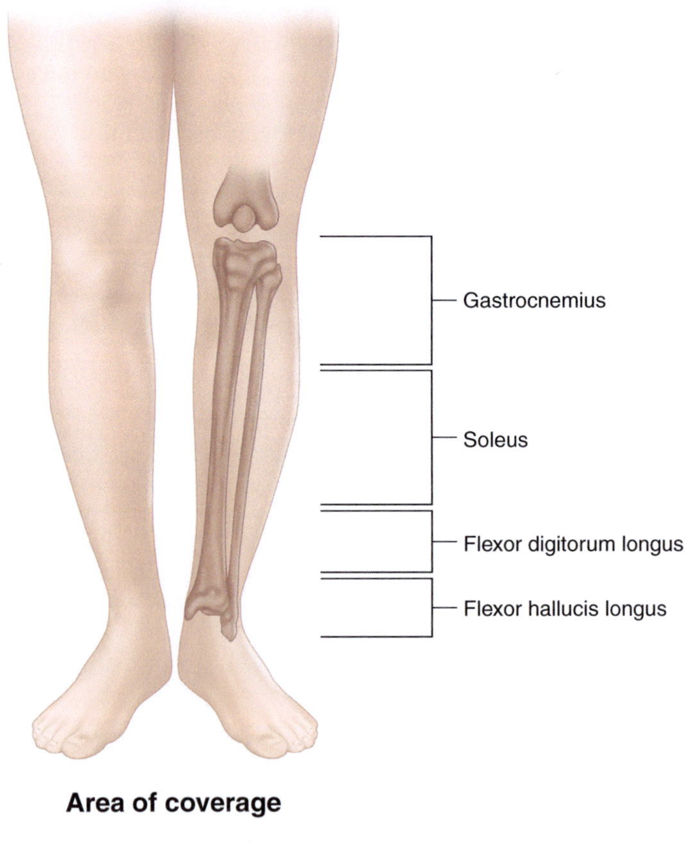

FIGURE 10.1 Areas of coverage. The lower leg can be divided into regions that are amenable to local muscle flap coverage

requires local fasciocutaneous flaps or free tissue transfers.

Adequate débridement of all devitalized tissue and bone is mandatory in preparation for coverage with all flaps. The success or failure of the flap depends on adequate débridement, especially when treating osteomyelitis [1].

Mathes and Nahai Muscle Classification

Figure 10.2 illustrates the circulatory patterns of muscle flaps in the Mathes and Nahai Classification [2]:

- ***Type I:*** A single vascular pedicle enters the muscle and is critical to flap survival. (Examples in lower extremity: tensor fascia lata, gastrocnemius, abductor digiti minimi)
- ***Type II:*** Dominant vascular pedicle, which is critical to survival of the flap, and minor vascular pedicles. Use of this type of flap generally requires division of all or some of the minor pedicles. (Examples: gracilis, rectus femoris, vastus medialis, vastus lateralis, vastus intermedialis, biceps femoris, semitendinosus, semimembranosus, soleus, abductor hallucis, peroneus longus, and peroneus brevis)
- ***Type III:*** Two dominant pedicles, either of which can support the entire muscle. (Example: gluteus maximus; none in the lower extremity)
- ***Type IV:*** Multiple segmental vascular pedicles, which are generally equal in size. Each segment of muscle is supported by its corresponding segmental pedicle. Typically, a division of two or more pedicles can support a portion of the muscle, but the muscle will not survive if an excessive number of pedicles are divided during flap elevation. (Examples: sartorius, flexor hallucis longus, flexor digitorum longus, tibialis posterior, extensor hallucis longus, extensor digitorum longus, tibialis anterior, peroneus tertius, plantaris, and popliteus)
- ***Type V:*** One dominant pedicle and secondary segmental pedicles. The dominant pedicle can reliably ensure survival of the muscle. The secondary vascular pedicles, which generally enter at the opposite end from the dominant pedicle,

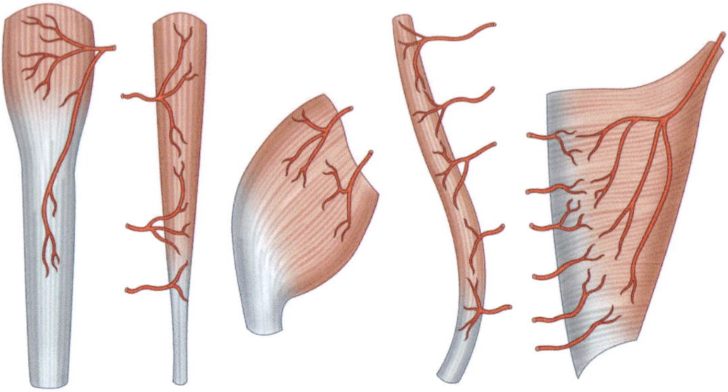

FIGURE 10.2 Mathes and Nahai classification of muscle flaps. A type I muscle has a single dominant pedicle. A type II muscle has a major and minor pedicle. Typically, the flap cannot survive on the minor pedicle alone. Type III muscle flaps have two dominant pedicles and can survive on either pedicle. A type IV muscle flap has multiple segmental pedicles. Each pedicle supplies blood flow to the adjacent muscle only. A type V muscle has one dominant pedicle and several minor pedicles. The muscle can survive on either the dominant pedicle or the minor pedicles

can also support the muscle if the dominant pedicle is divided. (Example: latissimus dorsi; none in the lower extremity)

Types I, III, and V have the most reliable vascularity. Types II and IV muscle flaps are less reliable because the vascular pedicle to the distal portion or segment of muscle must be divided to achieve an adequate arc of rotation to be useful for wound coverage. The upper leg muscles are all type II except for the tensor fascia lata (TFL, type I) and the sartorius (type IV). The lower leg muscles are mainly type IV except for the gastrocnemius (type I), peroneus longus (type II), peroneus brevis (type II), and soleus (type II) [2].

Pedicled Muscle Flap

The use of a pedicled muscle flap is based on the arc of rotation of the muscle from its neurovascular pedicle. The arc of rotation of the muscle is limited by the point of entry and length of the vascular pedicle. An estimation of the arc of rotation can be made with a laparotomy pad placed with one end at the base of the vascular pedicle and the other end defining the end of the usable muscle. This pad can then be rotated to ensure that the muscle flap can reach and cover the defect and can define the limits of coverage.

A muscle flap can be segmentally elevated, which can preserve function and decrease bulk at the recipient site. Type III muscles are ideal for segmental flaps because they have a dual supply. Type I and II muscles would need to be divided along the branches of the dominant pedicle. Type V muscles can be split or can be taken as a smaller flap. Type IV muscles require elevation in a segmental fashion, because the entire muscle will not survive off a single segmental pedicle.

These flaps can also be distally based, in which the dominant pedicle is divided and the flap is designed off the minor pedicles located opposite to the dominant pedicle. Generally, the entire muscle will not survive off the minor pedicle alone, so only a segment of muscles is elevated on a specific minor pedicle.

The muscle flap can be tunneled under a skin bridge and the surface skin grafted if exposed. Muscle flaps tend to be bulky in the acute setting, but with time the muscle will atrophy. If the neurovascular bundle is kept intact, however, then the muscle fibers will not atrophy in the same way as when the nerve has been divided. Following are some tips for the most common workhorse muscle flaps for coverage of the lower extremity.

Upper Leg

There are three compartments in the upper leg, housing a total of 14 muscles:

- The *anterior compartment* of the thigh contains the sartorius muscles and the four heads of the quadriceps (the

rectus femoris, vastus lateralis, vastus intermedius, and vastus medialis), along with the articularis genus. These muscles are supplied by the femoral nerve.
- The *adductor/medial compartment* of the thigh contains the adductor magnus, adductor longus, adductor brevis, gracilis, and pectineus. The medial compartment muscles are supplied by the obturator nerve.
- The *posterior compartment* contains the hamstring potion of the biceps femoris, semitendinosus, and semimembranosus muscles. The posterior muscles are supplied by the sciatic nerve.

The anterior thigh compartment is the source for most of the commonly used flaps (Fig. 10.3). The blood supply to the anterior compartment is predominantly from branches of the profunda femoris artery—the medial and lateral circumflex femoral branches. Typically, the medial circumflex is smaller than the lateral circumflex. It courses medially just deep to the adductor longus muscle, lying superficially on the adductor magnus muscle, and terminates into the gracilis muscle (a type II muscle) as the major vascular pedicle. The lateral circumflex femoral artery travels laterally and deep to the rectus femoris, giving two branches to the deep surface. It emerges at the lateral border of the rectus femoris deep to the sartorius muscle (type IV muscle). Then the vessel gives a descending branch to supply the vastus lateralis and continues laterally to give a small branch to the gluteus minimus muscle and two or three large terminal branches into the TFL (type I muscle).

Lower Leg

The muscles of the lower leg can be rotated to a variety of locations based on the specific muscle flap used (Fig. 10.4). The lower leg consists of four fascial compartments and 13 muscles:

- The *anterior compartment* contains the tibialis anterior, extensor hallucis longus, extensor digitorum longus, and peroneus tertius. The deep peroneal nerve and anterior tibial vessels are in the anterior compartment, but the

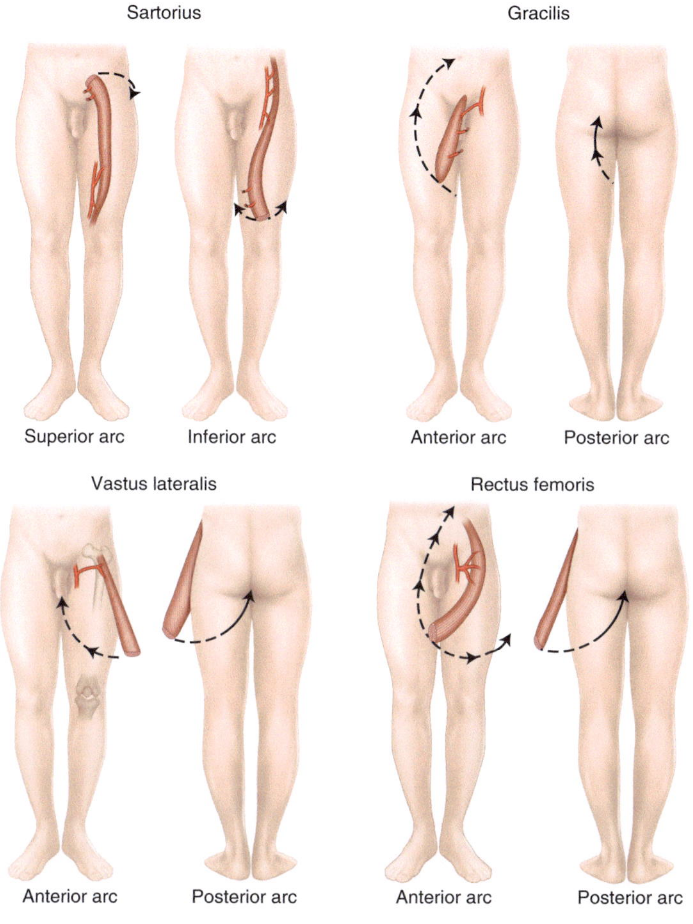

Figure 10.3 Upper leg arc of rotation. Multiple regions in the thigh can be covered by rotational muscle flaps. The figure shows the arc of rotation for the sartorius flap, the gracilis flap, the vastus lateralis flap, and the rectus femoris flap

common peroneal nerve first courses through the lateral compartment and contributes to the superficial peroneal nerve, which subsequently lies outside of the fascial envelope of the lateral compartment.

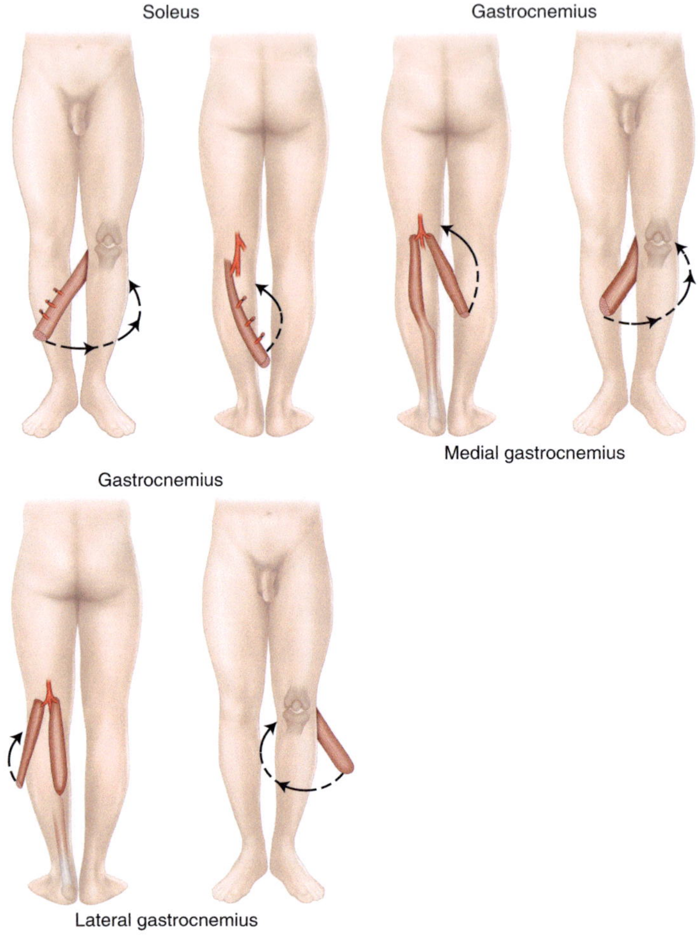

FIGURE 10.4 Lower leg arc of rotation. Multiple regions in the lower leg can be covered by rotational muscle flaps. The figure shows the arc of rotation for the soleus flap and the medial and lateral gastrocnemius flaps

- The *lateral compartment* contains the peroneus longus and peroneus brevis muscles. The peroneal artery is contained within the lateral compartment.
- The *posterior compartment* is divided into deep and superficial groups:

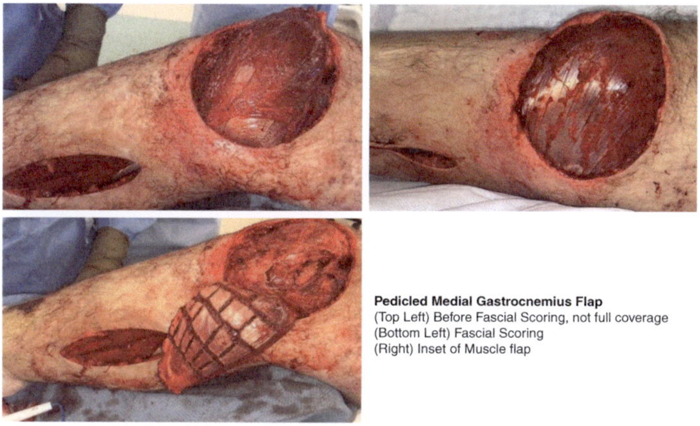

FIGURE 10.5 Pedicled gastrocnemius flap. These photos show a large defect of the knee and distal tibia (*top left*). A medial gastrocnemius flap is elevated and tunneled to close the defect. To provide full coverage, the muscle flap can be extended by scoring the fascia along the undersurface of the muscle (*bottom left, right*). The donor defect is closed primarily. The muscle is typically covered with a split-thickness skin graft to allow it to shrink into the defect

- The *deep posterior compartment* contains the tibialis posterior, flexor hallucis longus, flexor digitorum longus, and popliteus muscles. The tibial nerve and posterior tibial artery are contained within the deep posterior compartment.
- The *superficial posterior compartment* contains the gastrocnemius, soleus, and plantaris muscles.

The gastrocnemius and soleus are the most commonly used muscle flaps of the lower leg (Fig. 10.5). The gastrocnemius muscle (a type I muscle) is supplied by sural branches of the popliteal artery. The soleus muscle is a type II muscle. The posterior tibial artery is the dominant vascular pedicle and supplies the tibial origin of the muscle; the fibular origin is supplied by the peroneal artery. The flexor digitorum longus (type IV muscle) is supplied by branches of the posterior tibial artery. The flexor hallucis longus, also a type IV muscle, is supplied by branches of the peroneal artery [3–6].

References

1. Salgado CJ, Mardini S, Jamali AA, Ortiz J, Gonzales R, Chen HC. Muscle versus nonmuscle flaps in the reconstruction of chronic osteomyelitis defects. Plast Reconstr Surg. 2006;118:1401–11.
2. Mathes SJ, Nahai F. Classification of the vascular anatomy of muscles: experimental and clinical correlation. Plast Reconstr Surg. 1981;67:177–87.
3. Arnold PG, Mixter RC. Making the most of the gastrocnemius muscles. Plast Reconstr Surg. 1983;72:38–48.
4. Hallock GG, Morris SF. Skin grafts and local flaps. Plast Reconstr Surg. 2011;127:5e–22e.
5. Reddy V, Stevenson TR. MOC-PS(SM) CME Article: lower extremity reconstruction. Plast Reconstr Surg. 2008;121(4 Suppl):1–7.
6. Soltanian H, Garcia RM, Hollenbeck ST. Current concepts in lower extremity reconstruction. Plast Reconstr Surg. 2015;136:815e–29e.

Chapter 11
Soft Tissue Reconstruction of the Thigh

Trevor C. Hansen and Derek E. Bell

Goals of reconstruction for proximal lower extremity wounds vary according to the specific location, involved structures, and etiology of the index lesion. Commonly, the plastic surgeon is tasked with providing soft tissue for a traumatic or iatrogenic wound to cover vital vascular structures, fill large dead space, protect implants or hardware, or resurface areas prone to chronic pressure. Thankfully, the proximal lower extremity is uniquely suited to local tissue harvest, owing to several composite flap options with well-established vascular patterns and functional redundancy.

T. C. Hansen (✉) · D. E. Bell
Division of Plastic and Reconstructive Surgery, University of Rochester Medical Center, Rochester, NY, USA
e-mail: trevor_hansen@URMC.rochester.edu

S. T. Hollenbeck et al. (eds.), *Handbook of Lower Extremity Reconstruction*, https://doi.org/10.1007/978-3-030-41035-3_11

Thigh Anatomy and Function

Anatomically, the thigh can be separated into three compartments—the anterior, posterior, and medial compartments—which are encircled by investing fascia and extend longitudinally along the length of the femur. Functionally, the muscles in these compartments contribute to the core movements necessary for ambulation: knee extension (anterior), knee flexion (posterior), and leg adduction (medial).

The blood supply to the thigh is important, not only for supplying structures of the upper leg, but also for ensuring circulation to the entirety of the lower extremity. Entry of the femoral artery into the lower extremity occurs at the femoral triangle, bounded by the inguinal ligament superiorly, the adductor longus medially, and the sartorius muscle laterally. Given the easily identified anatomy, this area is often accessed for vascular procedures. After entering the thigh, the femoral artery gives off a deep branch, called the profunda femoris, which courses within the medial compartment and supplies branches to a majority of the medial and posterior muscles. Near the origin of the profunda femoris arise the medial and lateral circumflex arteries, which supply muscles of the medial and anterior compartments respectively. Other notable branches of the femoral artery include the superficial circumflex iliac artery and the medial descending genicular artery. Once the femoral artery passes through the adductor hiatus of the adductor magnus muscle just proximal to the knee, it becomes the popliteal artery and continues distally into the lower leg. Skin of the thigh is supplied via septocutaneous and musculocutaneous perforators from the above vessels.

Three main nerves traverse the thigh, one through each of the three muscle compartments. The femoral nerve passes under the inguinal ligament to enter the anterior compartment and supply innervation to the included muscles, as well as cutaneous branches to the overlying anterior thigh and knee skin. The obturator nerve enters the medial compartment through the obturator canal before branching to innervate the thigh adductors and supply cutaneous thigh sensation. The sciatic nerve is responsible for all posterior compartment muscles before continuing distally to become the common peroneal and tibial nerves. Finally, there is a direct branch of the lumbar plexus, the lateral femoral cutaneous nerve, which enters the anterior compartment laterally before piercing the tensor fascia lata and supplying cutaneous sensation to the anterolateral thigh.

Free Flaps Versus Local Flaps

Thigh defects vary widely in size and involved structures, depending on the etiology and chronicity of the wound. Despite their variability, however, most wounds can be treated with locoregional flaps alone, without the need for free tissue transfers, because the thigh comprises sufficient soft tissue options. Composite pedicled flaps may include a combination of skin, fascia, and muscle, depending on availability and reconstructive need. Though most vascular pedicles to thigh musculature enter proximally, recurrent distal circulation may be sufficient for certain flaps to allow for distally based rotation and therefore distal thigh and proximal leg coverage.

Local Flaps for the Hip

A substantial proportion of hip defects arise from poor pressure control in an otherwise immobile or insensate patient. Pressure ulcers can progress to include all subcutaneous structures and can be difficult to manage, given their potential for bacterial colonization or infection, as well as the need for pressure offloading. In these situations, consideration is given to providing well-vascularized soft tissue while minimizing donor site morbidity, as these wounds are often recalcitrant and require additional future procedures.

When more conservative methods, including negative-pressure wound therapy and skin grafting, are not an option, local musculocutaneous and fasciocutaneous options must be considered. The anterolateral thigh flap is a close, reliable flap that provides adequate healthy tissue pedicled proximally on the descending lateral femoral circumflex artery. Additionally, this flap includes a fascial component for joint capsule coverage if needed, and it can be jointly harvested with the vastus lateralis if more significant tissue loss is present, or if surgical removal of the proximal femur (a Girdlestone procedure) is deemed necessary [1, 2].

Further posterior, the gluteus maximus advancement flap allows for mobilization of the inferior border of this muscle without disruption of its origin or insertion; it can then be advanced into the defect to provide muscular coverage. The overlying skin is also advanced, and modifications including V-Y closure allow for additional dermal tension relief [3, 4].

Other authors advocate for utilization of the tensor fascia lata musculocutaneous flap, which can be rotated directly, or islandized and tunneled to the defect, potentially decreasing donor site morbidity [5]. Other methods of closure include large random-pattern skin-only advancement flaps, which have the added benefit of potential readvancement should the wound recur.

Local Flaps for Groin Reconstruction

Given the proximity of large-caliber vessels to the skin surface as they exit the femoral triangle, the groin has become a common access site for vascular procedures, but the result can be untoward complications that create large soft tissue defects, often with exposure of critical structures at the wound base. In these instances, the primary goal of reconstruction becomes vascular protection and elimination of dead space. Reconstructive flaps are chosen predominantly for their ability to adequately reach the defect with enough tissue bulk to provide robust coverage. For smaller defects, the sartorius muscle lies in close proximity and can be disinserted from its iliac crest origin and turned inferomedially [6]. It can also be transected and rotated proximally or used as a turnover flap (Fig. 11.1). Alternatively, a proximally based

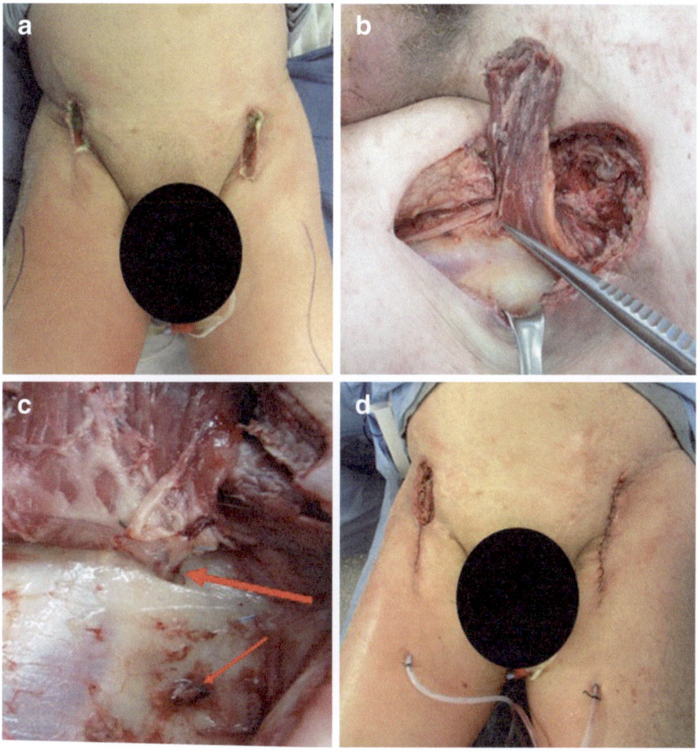

FIGURE 11.1 Sartorius flap for groin reconstruction. (**a**) The patient had bilateral groin wounds with exposed femoral arteries after endovascular aortic aneurysm repair. Reverse sartorius flaps were rotated to the bilateral groins. (**b**) Forceps identify the perforating branch of the superficial femoral artery. (**c**) The *large red arrow* identifies the perforating branch of the superficial femoral artery supplying the flaps; the *small red arrow* identifies a ligated branch necessary for sufficient rotation of the flap. (**d**) Final intraoperative result with closure of the skin over the left flap. The right side was left open and healed secondarily. (*Photos courtesy of* Derek Bell, MD)

gracilis flap, rotated about its main pedicle off the medial circumflex artery, may be used [7–9].

As the defect size increases, additional tissue must be mobilized. The rectus femoris flap, pedicled proximally off the lateral femoral circumflex artery, is an easily harvested muscle that supplies well-vascularized muscle bulk to the proximal groin with minimal functional morbidity [10, 11] (Fig. 11.2).

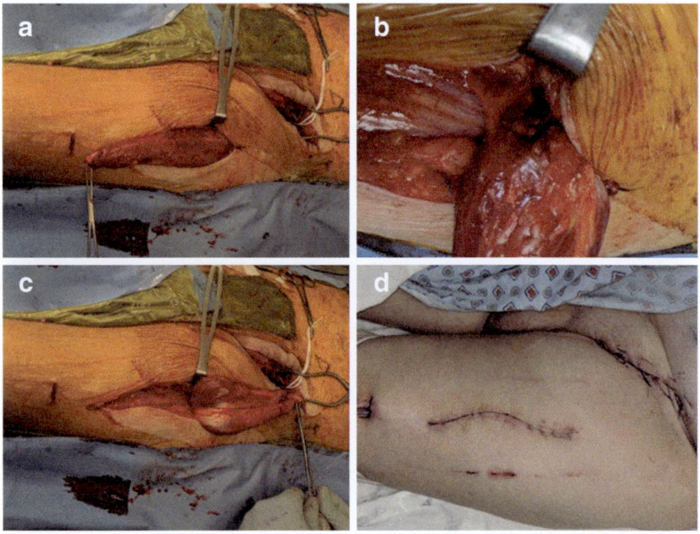

Figure 11.2 Left rectus femoris flap for groin coverage after femoral patch angioplasty infection and femoral artery rupture. (**a**) A lazy S incision is created over the mid-thigh, using the patella and anterior superior iliac spine as reference points along the trajectory of the flap. A small counter incision is created just proximal to the patella to access and transect the insertion of the rectus femoris tendon. (**b**) The descending branch of the lateral femoral circumflex artery pedicle entering the rectus femoris muscle. (**c**) The muscle flap is rotated and advanced proximally. It is passed deep to and through a subcutaneous tunnel. (**d**) Postoperative result shows a healed wound. (*Photos courtesy of* Derek Bell, MD)

For each of the above flaps, if there is not adequate skin for primary closure, a skin graft should be employed to cover exposed muscle. By contrast, a pedicled anterolateral thigh flap provides sufficient soft tissue for large wounds, including a fascial component as well as the underlying vastus lateralis muscle if needed, and the overlying skin paddle can be tailored to fit the groin defect prior to inset [12] (Fig. 11.3).

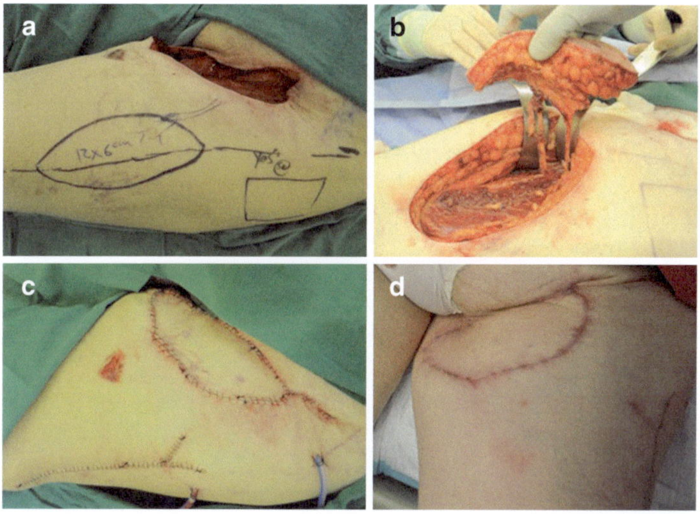

Figure 11.3 Left thigh pedicled anterolateral thigh (ALT) flap for groin coverage after skin cancer resection. (**a**) The patient had a resection of the soft tissue of the groin to remove a squamous cell carcinoma. The defect had exposed femoral vessels at the base. A pedicled ALT flap (12 × 6 cm) was designed to fill the defect. (**b**) The flap was elevated on two distinct perforators and tunneled under the rectus muscle. (**c**) The flap was inset to fill the defect, and the donor site was closed primarily. (**d**) The patient was seen 3 months after surgery, with a well-healed wound. (*Photos courtesy of* Scott T. Hollenbeck, MD)

Local Flaps for the Upper Knee

Knee and distal thigh defects offer a unique challenge, as the chosen donor tissue must offer enough bulk to fill the defect while remaining pliable and thin enough to cover a highly mobile joint surface. Additionally, medial and lateral defects cannot always be resurfaced by the same local tissue. The workhorse for knee defects remains the pedicled gastrocnemius muscle. Either the lateral or medial bellies of this muscle may be utilized, though the medial head is more commonly harvested, as it is larger, longer, and offers a longer pedicle around which to rotate. Additionally, the harvest of the lateral gastrocnemius muscle must contend with potential damage to the common peroneal nerve, which passes inferoposterior to the lateral head's origin [13].

When the gastrocnemius muscle is unavailable, the anterolateral thigh flap, with or without underlying vastus lateralis muscle, also serves as a reliable tissue source for reconstruction. This flap can be designed as a rotational flap, propeller flap, or transposition flap, depending on the location of the septocutaneous or musculocutaneous perforators [14, 15]. In most cases, the dominant pedicle to this flap, the descending branch of the lateral femoral circumflex artery, must be ligated, thereby causing the flap to rely on arborization through the lateral superior genicular artery distally. If needed, the flap may be delayed to ensure a more robust pedicle [13]. Other authors have advocated for salvage of complex knee wounds with distally pedicled gracilis [16] or sartorius [17] flaps, based on their minor or segmental pedicles respectively, but poor vascular reliability remains a potential pitfall.

Summary

Reconstruction of the thigh encompasses a vast breadth of wound sizes and etiologies, including trauma, infection, compression, iatrogenic wounds, and others. Thankfully, the thigh has a high number of available tissue options on reliable vascular pedicles that can be mobilized to provide adequate soft tissue coverage. Given the local options, free flaps are rarely required to bring new tissue to this area for wound coverage. Coverage in this area must be highly robust, however, for the reconstruction will likely be subject to repetitive compression or friction, may be covering critical vascular structures or stabilizing hardware, or may be placed over highly mobile joints.

References

1. Chang SH. Anterolateral thigh island pedicled flap in trochanteric pressure sore reconstruction. J Plast Reconstr Aesthet Surg. 2007;60:1074–5.
2. Rubayi S, Gabbay J, Kruger E, Ruhge K. The modified Girdlestone procedure with muscle flap for management of pressure ulcers and heterotopic ossification of the hip region in spinal injury patients: a 15-year review with long-term follow-up. Ann Plast Surg. 2016;77:645–52.
3. Nisanci M, Sahin I, Eski M, Alhan D. A new flap alternative for trochanteric pressure sore coverage: distal gluteus maximus musculocutaneous advancement flap. Ann Plast Surg. 2015;74:214–9.
4. Ricciardi BF, Henderson PW, McLawhorn AS, Westrich GH, Bostrom MP, Gayle LB. Gluteus maximus advancement flap procedure for reconstruction of posterior soft tissue deficiency in revision total hip arthroplasty. Orthopedics. 2017;40:e495–500.
5. Kim YH, Kim SW, Kim JT, Kim CY. Tensor fascia lata flap versus tensor fascia lata perforator-based island flap for the coverage of extensive trochanteric pressure sores. Ann Plast Surg. 2013;70:684–90.
6. Colwell AS, Donaldson MC, Belkin M, Orgill DP. Management of early groin vascular bypass graft infections with sartorius and rectus femoris flaps. Ann Plast Surg. 2004;52:49–53.
7. Shih PK, Cheng HT, Wu CI, Chang SC, Chen HC, Chen HH. Management of infected groin wounds after vascular surgery. Surg Infect. 2013;14:325–30.
8. Morasch MD, Sam AD, Kibbe MR, Hijjawi J, Dumanian GA. Early results with use of gracilis muscle flap coverage of infected groin wounds after vascular surgery. J Vasc Surg. 2004;39:1277–83.

9. Hussey AJ, Laing AJ, Regan PJ. An anatomical study of the gracilis muscle and its application in groin wounds. Ann Plast Surg. 2007;59:404–9.
10. Nelson JA, Fischer JP, Mackay DJ, Mirzabeigi MN, Cabiling DS, Kovach SJ, et al. The limited incision harvest of the rectus femoris flap for complex groin wound management. Ann Plast Surg. 2014;73:S161–4.
11. Sbitany H, Koltz PF, Girotto JA, Vega SJ, Langstein HN. Assessment of donor-site morbidity following rectus femoris harvest for infrainguinal reconstruction. Plast Reconstr Surg. 2010;126:933–40.
12. Fischer JP, Mirzabeigi MN, Sieber BA, Nelson JA, Wu LC, Kovach SJ, et al. Outcome analysis of 244 consecutive flaps for managing complex groin wounds. J Plast Reconstr Aesthet Surg. 2013;66:1396–404.
13. Rao AJ, Kempton SJ, Erickson BJ, Levine BR, Rao VK. Soft tissue reconstruction and flap coverage for revision total knee arthroplasty. J Arthroplast. 2016;31:1529–38.
14. Wong CH, Goh T, Tan BK, Ong YS. The anterolateral thigh perforator flap for reconstruction of knee defects. Ann Plast Surg. 2013;70:337–42.
15. Akhtar MS, Khan AH, Khurram MF, Ahmad I. Inferiorly based thigh flap for reconstruction of defects around the knee joint. Indian J Plast Surg. 2014;47:221–6.
16. Mitsala G, Varey AH, O'Neill JK, Chapman TW, Khan U. The distally pedicled gracilis flap for salvage of complex knee wounds. Injury. 2014;45:1776–81.
17. Clavert P, Cognet JM, Baley S, Stussi D, Prevost P, Babin SR, et al. Anatomical basis for distal sartorius muscle flap for reconstructive surgery below the knee. Anatomical study and case report. J Plast Reconstr Aesthet Surg. 2008;61:50–4.

Chapter 12
Knee and Proximal Lower Leg Wounds

Benjamin Googe, Somjade J. Songcharoen, and Peter B. Arnold

The primary goals for reconstruction of the knee and proximal leg include restoration of durable soft issue coverage and anatomical motion of the limb. Flap failure and the inability to achieve definitive soft tissue closure can lead to joint or hardware exposure and ultimately, amputation above the knee. As opposed to more distal lower extremity wounds, pedicled muscle flaps provide the workhorse for reconstruction [1].

Knee Anatomy and Function

The knee is a hinge joint formed by the distal femur and tibial plateau. Superficial to the joint is the patella, the largest sesamoid bone in the body. It communicates proximally with the extensor muscles of the thigh and inserts distally onto the tibial tuberosity via the patellar ligament, providing protection to the joint. Medially, the pes anserinus crosses the knee and inserts on the tibia just superficial to the medial collateral

B. Googe · S. J. Songcharoen · P. B. Arnold (✉)
Division of Plastic and Reconstructive Surgery, University of Mississippi Medical Center, Jackson, MS, USA
e-mail: parnold@umc.edu

S. T. Hollenbeck et al. (eds.), *Handbook of Lower Extremity Reconstruction*, https://doi.org/10.1007/978-3-030-41035-3_12

ligament (MCL). Lateral support comes from the lateral collateral ligament (LCL), which crosses the knee joint to insert on the tibia and the fibular head. Along with the MCL and LCL, the anterior cruciate ligament (ACL) and posterior cruciate ligament (PCL) provide support to the knee by preventing translation and rotational stress during flexion and extension.

The vascular supply of the leg is located in the popliteal fossa, originating from the popliteal artery, which is a continuation of the superficial femoral artery. The medial and lateral sural arteries arise from the popliteal artery to supply the gastrocnemius muscle, providing a basis for inflow to pedicled and free flaps in this area. As the popliteal artery courses distally, it gives off its first major terminal branch, the anterior tibial artery (ATA), at the inferior border of the popliteus muscle. The ATA courses distally in the anterior compartment just anterior to the intraosseous membrane. Just distal to the ATA takeoff, the popliteal artery divides again, giving rise to its other two terminal branches: the posterior tibial and peroneal arteries. Both run in the deep posterior compartment and supply the rest of the leg.

Muscle and Fasciocutaneous Flaps

Primary closure under tension—or skin grafting alone—is frequently inadequate for wounds surrounding the knee. The likelihood of hardware or joint exposure is high, posing an unacceptable risk to the limb. Several options for robust muscle and fasciocutaneous coverage exist in the region. Further, skin grafts can be placed concurrently over flaps when skin paddles fail to provide complete coverage.

The medial and lateral bellies of the gastrocnemius lie in the superficial posterior compartment of the leg. Each forms a type I Mathes and Nahai muscle flap that can be used to cover the knee. Most injuries can be managed with the medial gastrocnemius flap, based on the medial sural artery (Fig. 12.1). Measures to provide additional surface area

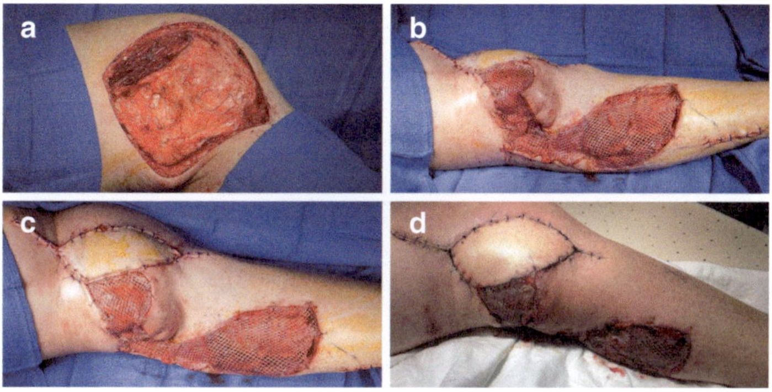

FIGURE 12.1 Medial gastrocnemius flap with skin paddle. (**a**) Soft tissue defect with exposed capsule. (**b**) Posterior view, donor defect with skin graft. (**c**) Lateral view of skin paddle. (**d**) 1 month postoperative

include disoriginating the flap at the medial femoral condyle, performing fascial scoring along the muscle belly, and extending the flap harvest distally to include a segment of the Achilles tendon [2].

The lateral gastrocnemius similarly can be used for distal thigh, knee, and proximal tibial soft tissue coverage, but it has some distinct differences from its medial counterpart (Fig. 12.2). It is based off the lateral sural artery and has a shorter muscle belly, and consequently, a smaller arc of rotation. Functional donor site morbidity is limited with flaps based on either muscle head. Most patients can expect near-complete recovery with compensation by other posterior compartment muscles [3].

Alternatively, if the defect requires only skin coverage, a fasciocutaneous flap based on the sural artery would provide adequate reconstruction at no functional cost. Although both medial and lateral perforator flaps have been described, the medial sural artery perforator (MSAP) flap is more robust and more commonly utilized. Fasciocutaneous perforator flaps can be raised as an advancement, propeller, or pedicled island flap [4].

The soleus muscle lies deep to the gastrocnemius and originates just distal to the medial head of the gastrocnemius

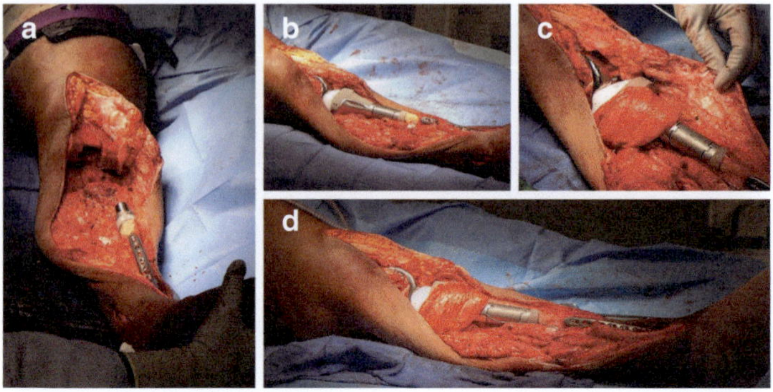

FIGURE 12.2 Lateral gastrocnemius flap. (**a**) Large bony and soft tissue defect. The flap was raised with joint hardware disarticulated to provide excellent exposure. (**b**) Knee prosthesis in place. (**c**) Lateral gastrocnemius flap covering prosthesis. (**d**) Lateral view of coverage. The skin was closed primarily

muscle. Although it is best suited for soft tissue coverage of the middle third of the tibia [5, 6], it can also be used for soft tissue coverage of the knee, either alone or in conjunction with a medial gastrocnemius flap for large defects. It is a type II Mathes and Nahai flap, with arterial supply from the popliteal artery proximally, and branches from the peroneal and tibial vessels distally [7–9]. Variations of the flap include the hemisoleus, which may limit postoperative functional defects, and a reverse-flow flap based distally for distal wounds. The utility of the reverse soleus flap is limited, however, as the blood supply is tenuous and tends to be located in the zone of injury for traumatic wounds.

The reverse pedicled anterolateral thigh (ALT) flap is a robust pedicled fasciocutaneous flap with a dissection pattern familiar to those accustomed to free tissue transfer. The main pedicle receives blood supply from the descending branch of the lateral femoral circumflex (LFC) artery, which also receives distal flow from genicular artery branches around the knee. Pedicle length is maximized by choosing a more proximal perforator for the skin paddle. In order to avoid flap failure, adequate retrograde flow may be confirmed by pre-clamping the

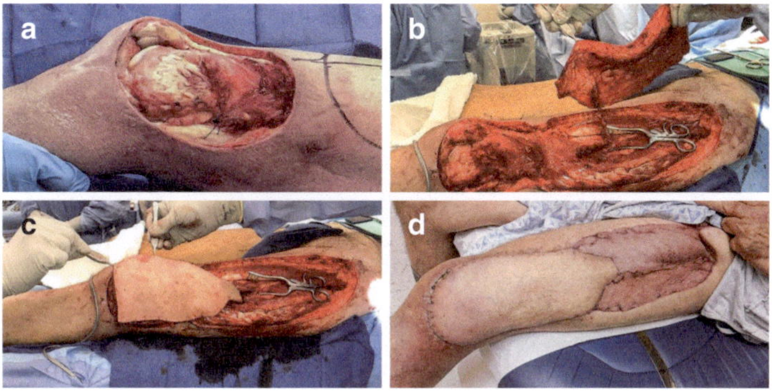

FIGURE 12.3 Anterolateral thigh fasciocutaneous propeller flap. (**a**) Lateral soft tissue defect. (**b**) Large skin paddle on a proximal perforator. (**c**) Initial inset with some intraoperative flap ischemia; a decision was made to delay the flap. (**d**) 3 months postoperative

LFC artery and vein to assess distal perfusion and outflow. It is prudent to have a low threshold for flap delay (Fig. 12.3) [10]. Delay incorporates the concepts of improving perfusion to the flap by dividing the dominant blood supply to the flap in order to allow the secondary circulatory contributions to increase their contribution to nourishing the flap [11]. While outside the scope of this chapter, it is felt that there are multiple different ways the delay phenomenon positively contributes to improving perfusion in flaps as early as 4 hours after vessel division and up to weeks where neovascularization occurs [12].

Other techniques include distally based gracilis or sartorius flaps for soft tissue defects of the knee [3, 7, 13].

Free Tissue Transfer

In some circumstances, local reconstructive options can be limited, necessitating free tissue transfer for definitive coverage. Options include the ALT, latissimus dorsi, and gracilis, among others. Selection of the flap should be based on the defect characteristics, with consideration given to the pedicle length necessary for tension-free inset [14]. Recipient vessels include the anterior and posterior tibial arteries, sural arteries, or genicular arteries. Anastomosis to recipient vessels should take place outside the zone of injury, utilizing vein grafts or arteriovenous loops when indicated.

Injuries of the Extensor Mechanism

Complex injuries to the knee can extend beyond the bony and ligamentous framework. Injury to the patella and extensor mechanism present a unique challenge to the reconstructive surgeon. Failure to reconstruct these structures can result in salvage arthrodesis or even amputation. The use of allografts for this purpose has become more popular, but we prefer autologous reconstruction with the gastrocnemius. The flap provides soft tissue coverage of the joint and bridges the tendinous defect in the extensor apparatus. Good clinical outcomes have been reported both anecdotally and in retrospective studies [15]. Techniques are similar to elevation for other reasons, but the aponeurosis must be preserved in order to provide strength to the extensor repair. Therefore, extensive scoring must be avoided. When additional length is needed, the muscle can be disoriginated from the femoral condyle. Either of the gastrocnemius muscle heads may be used, but we prefer the medial head for reconstruction, when it is available.

Postoperative Care and Complications

Rehabilitation can be a long course for patients after lower extremity reconstruction. Advances in orthopedics and internal fixation have allowed for earlier mobilization. After reconstruction, motion of the knee joint should be limited by a brace or knee immobilizer for 2–4 weeks, followed by range-of-motion exercises with physical therapy. Attention to strap placement is paramount, as unwanted pressure across flap pedicles can result in congestion and ischemia. Wound dehiscence and infection can also result in flap failure and potential loss of limb salvage. A high index of clinical suspicion and early intervention with antibiotics and débridement help avoid hardware and joint exposure.

Summary

The knee joint plays a crucial role in physiologic ambulation. With reconstruction, providing durable soft tissue coverage of the joint and any hardware in the region is essential. Careful coordination with orthopedics is key in our practice. Having a clear understanding of functional anatomy and reconstructive goals helps direct the appropriate selection of pedicled or free flaps in order to obtain optimal results and, ultimately, limb salvage.

References

1. Armstrong MB, editor. Lower extremity trauma. New York: Informa Health Care; 2007.
2. Walton Z, Armstrong M, Traven S, Leddy L. Pedicled rotational medial and lateral gastrocnemius flaps: surgical technique. J Am Acad Orthop Surg. 2017;25:744–51.
3. Kramers-de Quervain IA, Läuffer JM, Käch K, Trentz O, Stüssi E. Functional donor-site morbidity during level and uphill gait after a gastrocnemius or soleus muscle-flap procedure. J Bone Joint Surg Am. 2001;83:239–46.
4. Mohan AT, Sur YJ, Zhu L, Morsy M, Wu PS, Moran SL, et al. The concepts of propeller, perforator, keystone, and other local flaps and their role in the evolution of reconstruction. Plast Reconstr Surg. 2016;138:710e–29e.
5. Soltanian H, Garcia RM, Hollenbeck ST. Current concepts in lower extremity reconstruction. Plast Reconstr Surg. 2015;136:815e–29e.
6. Lachica RD. Evidence-based medicine: management of acute lower extremity trauma. Plast Reconstr Surg. 2017;139:287e–301e.

7. Gravvanis A, Kyriakopoulos A, Kateros K, Tsoutsos D. Flap reconstruction of the knee: a review of current concepts and a proposed algorithm. World J Orthop. 2014;5:603–13.
8. Hyodo I, Nakayama B, Takahashi M, Toriyama K, Kamei Y, Torii S. The gastrocnemius with soleus bi-muscle flap. Br J Plast Surg. 2004;57:77–82.
9. Mathes SJ, Nahai F. Vascular anatomy of muscle: classification and application. In: Mathes SJ, Nahai F, editors. Clinical applications for muscle and musculocutaneous flaps. St. Louis: Mosby; 1982. p. 87.
10. Bekarev M, Goch AM, Geller DS, Garfein ES. Distally based anterolateral thigh flap: an underutilized option for peripatellar wound coverage. Strategies Trauma Limb Reconstr. 2018;13:151–62.
11. Dhar SC, Taylor GI. The delay phenomenon: the story unfolds. Plast Reconstr Surg. 1999;104:2079–91.
12. Taylor GI, Corlett RJ, Caddy CM, Zelt RG. An anatomic review of the delay phenomenon. II. Clinical applications. Plast Reconstr Surg. 1992;89:408–16, discussion 417–8.
13. Ling BM, Wettstein R, Staub D, Schaefer DJ, Kalbermatten DF. The medial sural artery perforator flap: the first choice for soft-tissue reconstruction about the knee. J Bone Joint Surg Am. 2018;100:211–7.
14. Fang T, Zhang EW, Lineaweaver WC, Zhang F. Recipient vessels in the free flap reconstruction around the knee. Ann Plast Surg. 2013;71:429–33.
15. Jepegnanam TS, Boopalan PR, Nithyananth M, Titus VT. Reconstruction of complete knee extensor mechanism loss with gastrocnemius flaps. Clin Orthop Relat Res. 2009;467:2662–7.

Chapter 13
Soft Tissue Reconstruction of the Middle Third of the Leg

Katherine C. Benedict and Benjamin McIntyre

The tibia is one of the strongest bones in the body, but ironically, its anterior surface is covered by an extremely thin layer of soft tissue that is easily devascularized. Injuries to this part of the leg are high-energy, frequently resulting in comminution of both the tibia and fibula. Concomitant soft tissue degloving and necrosis are the norm. Goals of reconstruction at this level include durable coverage of open fractures or denuded bone in order to achieve reliable bone fixation and healing before osteomyelitis can set in. Aesthetically pleasing results in this area can be difficult, and in many instances a decision must be made to sacrifice some function of the limb in order to preserve the limb. In this high-stakes area, failure to adequately provide appropriate soft tissue coverage can result in non-union, mal-union, osteomyelitis, and eventual limb loss. For certain injuries, pedicled muscle flaps in the middle third of the leg can be used as an initial modality for

K. C. Benedict · B. McIntyre (✉)
Division of Plastic and Reconstructive Surgery, University of Mississippi Medical Center, Jackson, MS, USA
e-mail: bmcintyre@umc.edu

S. T. Hollenbeck et al. (eds.), *Handbook of Lower Extremity Reconstruction*, https://doi.org/10.1007/978-3-030-41035-3_13

the reconstructive surgeon. More devastating injuries or multilevel injuries will likely require free tissue transfer to achieve soft tissue coverage.

Leg Anatomy and Function

Thorough knowledge of anatomy at this level is paramount when making useful decisions regarding flap options at the level of the mid tibia. There are four muscular compartments: the anterior, lateral, superficial posterior, and deep posterior compartments. In this region, most of these muscles are bulky and not tendinous. The Achilles tendon begins at the very lower end of this region. Distally, beyond the musculotendinous junctions of these compartmental muscles, little to no muscular soft tissue coverage is available, and this affects the arc of rotation when choosing a local flap.

The primary blood supply to the leg arises from the femoral artery, which becomes the popliteal artery after its passage through the adductor hiatus. After traversing the popliteal fossa, it branches into the anterior tibial artery, posterior tibial artery, and peroneal artery. These three arteries, accompanied by their venae comitantes, provide the blood supply to the leg and foot. With severe fractures, one or more of these vessels may be injured. Knowledge of the location and continuity of these vessels is imperative, as they may be a donor vessel for a free flap or may be the main blood supply to a pedicled muscle flap.

The muscles of the leg are innervated by three major motor nerves, which arise as terminal branches of the sciatic nerve. The anterior compartment is innervated by the deep peroneal nerve and receives its arterial supply from the anterior tibial artery. The lateral compartment is innervated by the superficial peroneal nerve and is the vascular territory of the peroneal artery. Finally, the superficial and deep posterior compartments are innervated by the posterior tibial nerve, with blood supply from the posterior tibial artery. These compartments are separated by distinct intermuscular septa. Damage to the common peroneal nerve results in foot drop and loss of foot eversion with dorsal foot anesthesia. Damage to the deep branch of the peroneal nerve results in

Table 13.1 Gustilo-Anderson classification of open fractures classification

	Description
Grade I	Open fracture with clean wound <1 cm
Grade II	Open fracture with laceration >1 cm but no significant soft-tissue loss, avulsion, or flap
Grade IIIA	High-energy trauma causing open fracture; or open fracture with extensive soft-tissue laceration or flaps and adequate soft-tissue coverage
Grade IIIB	Open fracture with extensive soft-tissue injury loss with periosteal stripping and bone exposure; often with massive contamination
Grade IIIC	Open fracture with arterial injury requiring repair

From Gustilo et al. [1]; with permission

foot drop and anesthesia of the first web space. Damage to the superficial branch results in loss of foot eversion and anesthesia of the dorsal foot.

A comprehensive evaluation must include vascular examination for palpable pulses and Doppler signals, evaluation of motor function of all compartments of the leg, and preoperative sensory evaluation to determine deficits. Examination of radiographs can also assist in decision-making regarding reconstructive options. Accomplished reconstructive surgeons will possess a solid background in the fundamentals of fracture fixation at this level. It is also best to develop a multispecialty team approach when confronting patients with these injuries. Familiarity with the Gustilo classification system of open fractures is paramount (Table 13.1). Definition of open fracture subtypes allows for differentiation of prognosis and treatment, as well as the likelihood of complications and eventual amputation.

Muscle and Fasciocutaneous Flaps

Just as the gastrocnemius flap is the workhorse of proximal third fractures, the soleus muscle flap should be the surgeon's "go-to" pedicled muscle flap for middle third tibial

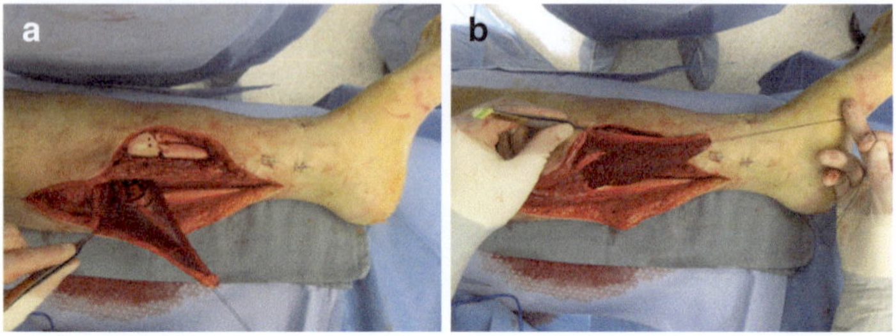

Figure 13.1 Soleus flap. (**a**) Limited mid-tibial wound with exposed plate. (**b**) Demonstration of the arc of rotation of the soleus muscle flap

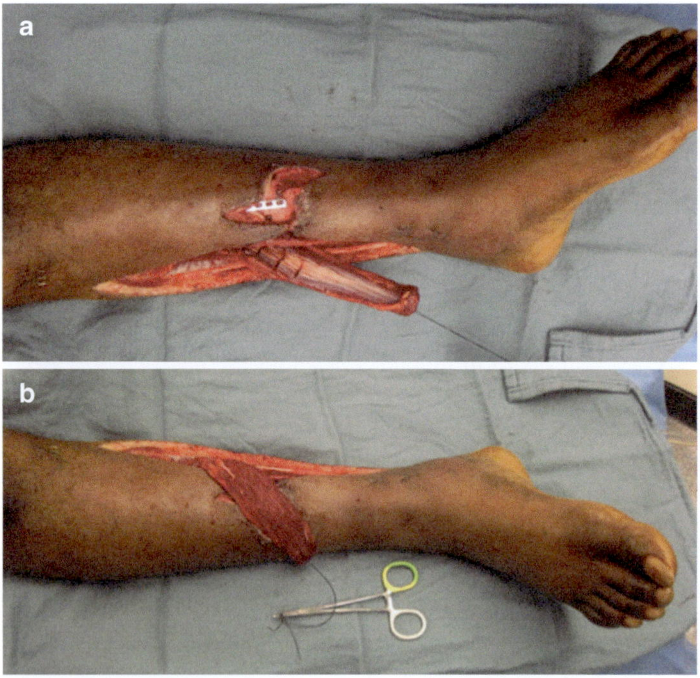

Figure 13.2 Soleus flap. (**a**) Comminuted tibial fracture with skin loss and flap dissected. (**b**) Demonstration of the arc of rotation of the soleus muscle flap

wounds (Figs. 13.1 and 13.2). The soleus muscle is wide and robust, with a reliable blood supply and a generous arc of rotation. Anatomically, the soleus muscle lies deep to the gastrocnemius and originates distal to the medial gastrocnemius muscle [2, 3]. It is a type II Mathes and Nahai flap, with arterial supply arising from the popliteal artery and its branches and its dominant blood supply entering proximally [4]. Variations of the flap include the hemisoleus, which may diminish postoperative functional limitations, or a reverse-flow, distally based flap for distal wounds. Use of the reverse soleus flap is limited because of its less-than-reliable blood supply and zone of injury implications in the trauma setting.

It is worth mentioning the gastrocnemius muscle in discussing reconstruction of the middle third of the leg. It is often used in injuries of the proximal third of the leg, but it also has limited utility in coverage of defects of the middle third. As a type I Mathes and Nahai muscle, the medial and lateral heads of the gastrocnemius muscle are supplied by the medial and lateral sural arteries, which branch from the popliteal artery just distal to the popliteal fossa [4]. Harvest of this flap results in minimal impairment of function while providing a reliable option for soft tissue coverage [5].

Lastly, the tibialis anterior muscle can be considered as a flap option for limited defects of the tibia in the patient with scarce other options for reconstruction and in whom foot dorsiflexion is no longer possible, or when the ankle is fused. This muscle lies in the anterior compartment of the leg, lateral to the tibia and medial to the extensor hallucis longus and extensor digitorum longus. It is a type IV Mathes and Nahai flap with arterial supply from 8 to 12 segmental pedicles arising from the anterior tibial artery or anterior recurrent vessels [6]. This muscle is the primary dorsiflexor of the foot, with an additional role in foot inversion. This muscle should never be taken in its entirety for soft tissue coverage [7].

Perforator Flaps for the Medial Third of the Leg

Reproducible dissection of perforators in the leg allows for reconstruction of soft tissue defects with limitation of donor site morbidity. Anterior tibial perforators lie between the tibia and tibialis anterior, and between the extensor digitorum longus and peroneus longus. The majority of perforators from all three vessels of the leg can be found in the intermuscular septa in three primary locations: 4–9 cm, 13–18 cm, and 21–26 cm from the intermalleolar line [8]. Perforator flaps are supplied by vessels originating from the deep vascular system and coursing through muscle or an intermuscular septum to reach the flap. These flaps are constructed either as advancement flaps (through linear tissue movement to cover the defect) or as propeller flaps (by means of rotatory movement of up to 180 degrees) [9].

A reverse, distally based sural artery flap is an excellent option for distal leg injuries, or a proximally based fasciocutaneous or adipofascial flap based on the superficial sural artery can provide a thin, sensate flap with minimal donor site morbidity. The pedicle is identified in the popliteal fossa, where the superficial sural artery branches from the popliteal artery. Because of its considerable pedicle length, this flap can be used for injuries about the knee, as well as for soft tissue defects of the middle third of the leg. Inclusion of the lesser saphenous vein within the pedicle of the flap decreases the risk of venous congestion and subsequent necrosis.

Propeller flaps, or local island fasciocutaneous flaps, are based on dissected perforators and can provide reliable soft tissue coverage in the middle third of the leg with negligible donor site morbidity. The design of these flaps involves arrangement of a larger and a smaller fasciocutaneous flap with the identified perforator located at the pivot point between these flaps. Rotation is then performed to fill the defect, with a maximum pedicle rotation arc of 180°. In consideration of skin paddle location, one must plan the donor flap away from critical structures such as the tibia, which cannot be closed primarily or skin-grafted [10].

Free Tissue Transfer

Free tissue transfer is a common solution for open tibia fractures of the middle third of the leg, particularly when there are multilevel injuries spanning the proximal and distal thirds of the tibia or when circumferential injuries are present. Powerful options exist that provide well-vascularized, bulky muscle for coverage (gracilis, rectus abdominus, latissimus dorsi). Many of these flaps have long pedicles that enable far-reaching applications. Free functional gracilis muscle transfer may also allow for limited restoration of foot dorsiflexion when utilized as a neurotized flap. The omental free flap (Fig. 13.3) is an excellent option given its lengthy pedicle, limited donor site morbidity when harvested laparoscopically, and the innate ability of the omentum to fight infection.

Work-up for patients prior to free tissue transfer includes evaluation of blood supply to the distal leg to ensure a minimum of one vessel run-off to the foot for adequate perfusion to the foot postoperatively. CT angiography should be considered in all patients with an open tibia fracture who are likely to undergo free flap reconstruction. Determination of which vessel to choose as recipient is dependent on the individual

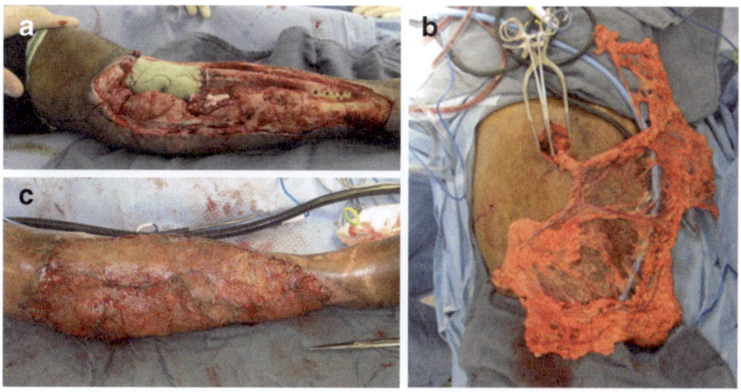

FIGURE 13.3 Omentum free flap. (**a**) Multilevel open tibia fracture with bone gap and antibiotic spacer. (**b**) Laparoscopically raised omentum flap. (**c**) Omentum flap inset with skin graft

patient's zone of injury and the location of the soft tissue defect. When performing a tibial-level free flap, it is imperative that all recipient vessels are well out of the zone of injury.

Summary

Lower extremity reconstruction is considered in terms of the proximal third, middle third, and distal third of the leg. Coverage of vital structures and restoration of patient function remains the primary goal of lower extremity reconstruction. The initial choice in the armamentarium of the plastic surgeon is often a pedicled muscle flap, including the soleus flap, tibialis anterior flap, and medial or lateral gastrocnemius flap, but local perforator flaps, propeller flaps, and free tissue transfer remain helpful options for patients with difficult soft tissue deficits.

References

1. Gustilo RB, Mendoza RM, Williams DN. Problems in the management of type III (severe) open fractures: a new classification of type III open fractures. J Trauma. 1984;24:742–6.
2. Soltanian H, Garcia RM, Hollenbeck ST. Current concepts in lower extremity reconstruction. Plast Reconstr Surg. 2015;136:815e–29e.
3. Lachica RD. Evidence-based medicine: management of acute lower extremity trauma. Plast Reconstr Surg. 2017;139:287e–301e.
4. Mathes SJ, Nahai F. Vascular anatomy of muscle: classification and application. In: Mathes SJ, Nahai F, editors. Clinical application for muscle and musculocutaneous flaps. St. Louis: Mosby; 1982. p. 87.
5. Abd-Almoktader MA. Gastrocnemius muscle flap for middle third leg defects. Egypt J Plast Reconstr Surg. 2014;38:197–204.
6. Mathes SJ, Nahai F. Tibialis anterior flap. In: Mathes SJ, Nahai F, editors. Reconstructive surgery: principles, anatomy, and techniques. New York: Churchill Livingstone; 1997. p. 1501–12.
7. Panse N, Sahasrabudhe P, Pande G, Chandanwale A, Dhongde R, Rajpal L. The split tibialis anterior muscle flap - a simple solu-

tion for longitudinal middle third tibial defects. Indian J Plast Surg. 2012;45:53–7.
8. Schaverien M, Saint-Cyr M. Perforators of the lower leg: analysis of perforator locations and clinical application for pedicled perforator flaps. Plast Reconstr Surg. 2008;122:161–70.
9. Dancey A, Blondeel PN. Technical tips for safe perforator vessel dissection applicable to all perforator flaps. Clin Plast Surg. 2010;37:593–606.
10. Teo TC. The propeller flap concept. Clin Plast Surg. 2010;37:615–26, vi.

Chapter 14
Soft Tissue Reconstruction of the Distal Third of the Lower Extremity

Roger W. Cason, Jonah P. Orr, and Suhail K. Mithani

Wounds of the distal third of the lower leg pose significant challenges for reconstructive surgeons. The paucity of local tissue limits local flap options, favoring the use of free tissue transfer. Additional factors, such as degree of local injury, vascular insult, and co-morbid conditions, often guide surgical decision-making. Regardless of the modality, reconstructive goals remain the same: achievement of stable wound coverage without impeding functionality.

R. W. Cason (✉) · J. P. Orr · S. K. Mithani
Division of Plastic, Maxillofacial, and Oral Surgery,
Duke University Health System, Durham, NC, USA
e-mail: roger.cason@duke.edu

S. T. Hollenbeck et al. (eds.), *Handbook of Lower Extremity Reconstruction*, https://doi.org/10.1007/978-3-030-41035-3_14

Relevant Surgical Anatomy of the Lower Leg

A thorough understanding of critical structures in this region is crucial in planning and executing a successful reconstruction. The reconstructive surgeon should be familiar with the locations of the three source arteries (peroneal, posterior tibial, and anterior tibial), which can serve as recipient vessels during microvascular anastomosis or can form the source vessel of a local perforator flap. In addition, venous drainage and innervation should be understood, particularly the greater and lesser saphenous veins and the sural, peroneal, and tibial nerves.

The anterior tibial artery (AT) resides in the anterior compartment and courses along the superficial surface of the interosseous membrane between the tibialis anterior and the extensor digitorum longus tendons (Fig. 14.1). At the level of the extensor retinaculum, the AT passes under the extensor hallucis longus (EHL) tendon to cross the ankle immediately lateral to the EHL, where it becomes the dorsalis pedis artery. It is typically accompanied by two venae comitantes. The deep peroneal nerve lies immediately medial to the AT in the

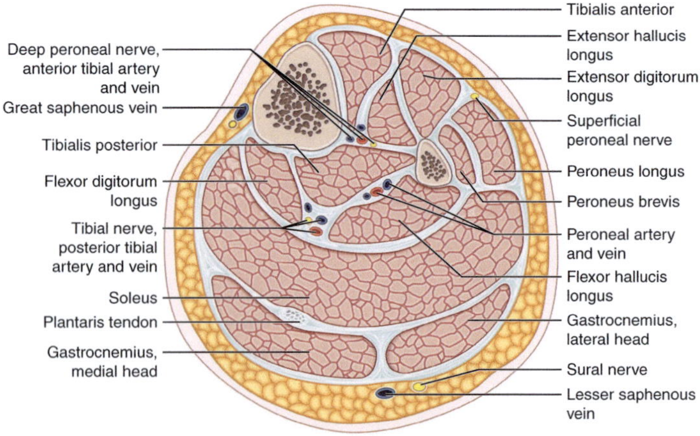

Figure 14.1 Cross-sectional anatomy of the distal lower extremity

distal leg. The posterior tibial artery (PT) is found between the superficial and deep posterior compartments. It courses medially and superficially as it descends, eventually accompanied by the tibial nerve and tendons of the tibialis posterior, flexor hallucis longus, and flexor digitorum longus as they pass posterior to the medial malleolus. The peroneal artery courses in the deep posterior compartment and is closely associated with the periosteum of the fibula. At the distal end of the fibula, the peroneal artery divides into the anterior lateral malleolar and lateral calcaneal arteries.

The great and lesser saphenous veins are the largest named vessels providing venous return of the lower extremity. The great saphenous vein originates on the dorsum of the foot and courses proximally along the extremity on its anteromedial surface, medial to the tibia. The lesser saphenous vein originates more laterally on the dorsum of the foot, runs posterior to the lateral malleolus, and courses superficially on the posterolateral aspect of leg with the sural nerve.

The sural nerve originates at the level of the mid-calf; it comprises a confluence of terminal branches of the tibial and common peroneal nerves. It runs superficially along the posterior aspect of the lateral malleolus and provides sensation to the skin of the distal and posterolateral leg, ankle, and foot. In addition to the sural nerve, the saphenous and superficial peroneal nerves make up the majority of the cutaneous innervation of the distal leg, providing anteromedial and posterolateral sensation, respectively. The tibial nerve provides plantar sensation to the foot and instep. As muscle innervation occurs more proximally in the leg, corresponding nerves contribute a more sensory role in the distal third of the lower leg.

Free Flaps Versus Local Flaps

Once a limb has been deemed salvageable and appropriate for flap reconstruction, a conversation between surgeon and patient must be had to assess the functional demands, goals, and expectations of the patient. Though a local flap may sound to the patient like the more attractive option, it is not always the appropriate solution, particularly in the distal leg. Although the advent of pedicled perforator flaps has spawned a rise in the usage of local flaps, free flaps remain the predominant option in this region [1]. Choice is dictated by the size and mechanism of the defect, patient co-morbidities, and in some cases, surgeon preference. Local flaps are typically limited by their small size, given the lack of available local and regional tissue for transfer. Larger defects or those with extensive local injury, as can be seen in high-energy trauma or as a sequela of prior radiation, are still best suited for free tissue transfer, which permits recruitment of healthy, well-vascularized tissue that can conform to difficult defects and maximize healing potential. Whichever method is chosen, the flap should match the defect in size and provide contour that does not interfere with the function of this important region, allowing for clothing and shoes and facilitating comfortable ambulation.

Local and Regional Flaps

Local flaps allow replacement of "like-with-like" tissue, shorter operative times, and containment of the donor site within the vicinity of the wound. Use is generally limited to smaller wounds, or to patients who cannot tolerate the prolonged anesthesia required for a free flap. The integrity of the surrounding local tissue must be ensured, as the transfer of tissue that is already of poor quality will result in an unstable reconstruction. Commonly employed local options that have utility in the distal third of the lower leg are bipedicled, reverse sural, and pedicled perforator flaps. Local muscle flaps are limited in this region, and should not be considered "workhorse" flaps.

The bipedicled flap (Fig. 14.2) is an example of a random pattern flap that is technically easy to perform and can achieve reasonable results for small defects, particularly those with minimal local tissue inflammation. Because it is a random pattern flap, and thus has no defined axial pedicle,

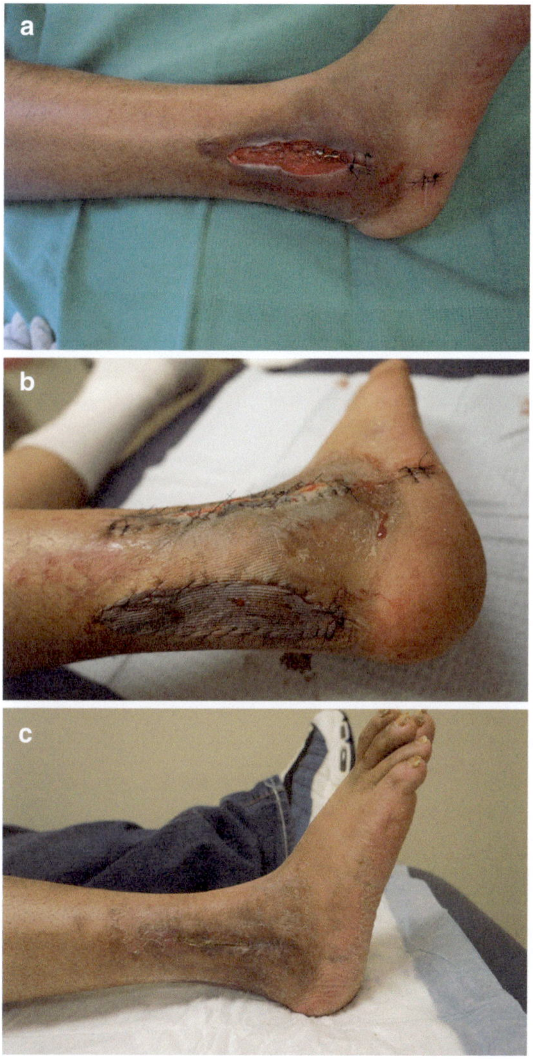

Figure 14.2 Bipedicled flap. (**a**) Débridement of local skin necrosis after open reduction and internal fixation of a bimalleolar fracture left this patient with a defect at the lateral malleolus measuring 7 × 2 cm. (**b**) A bipedicled flap of 8 × 5 cm was designed and advanced to cover the hardware. A split-thickness skin graft was used to resurface the donor defect. (**c**) Stable coverage of the hardware is demonstrated at 6 months postoperatively

strategic operative planning can ensure successful execution. Designing the flap 2–4 cm longer than the defect, at least 5 cm wide, and limiting undermining only to what is needed for sufficient mobility, will maximize perfusion [2]. For slightly larger defects, dual bipedicled flaps can be designed medially and laterally, and advanced toward the defect. Primary closure of the donor site is rarely possible; it usually requires skin grafting. Typical applications include coverage of small defects of the heel, lateral ankle, or pretibial area.

The reverse sural flap (Fig. 14.3) is a distally based flap that can be applied to the distal third and foot. It is a fasciocutaneous or adipocutaneous flap that relies on retrograde flow through the median superficial sural artery from the peroneal artery perforators at the posterolateral ankle. It receives additional vascular contributions from posterior tibial perforators, as well as venocutaneous perforators of the lesser saphenous vein and neurocutaneous perforators of the sural nerve [3, 4].

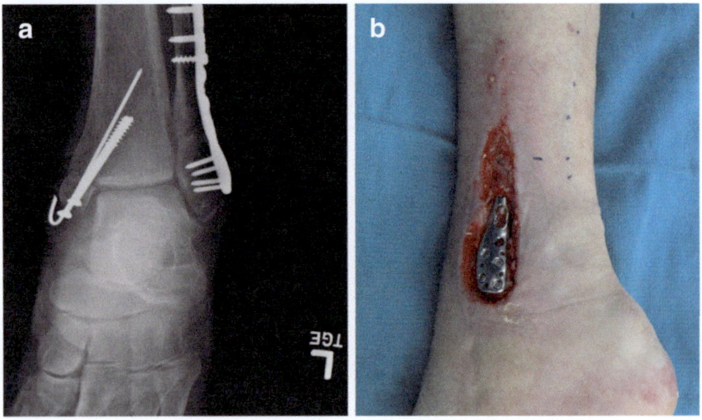

Figure 14.3 Reverse sural flap. (**a**) This patient underwent open reduction and internal fixation of a bimalleolar fracture. (**b**) Healing was complicated by cellulitis, skin necrosis, and exposed hardware at the lateral malleolus. After thorough débridement, the resultant wound measured 4 × 8 cm. (**c**) A 4 × 8 cm skin paddle was designed at the posterolateral calf. (**d**) This was elevated as a fasciocutaneous flap and rotated into the defect. (*Courtesy of* Detlev Erdmann, MD)

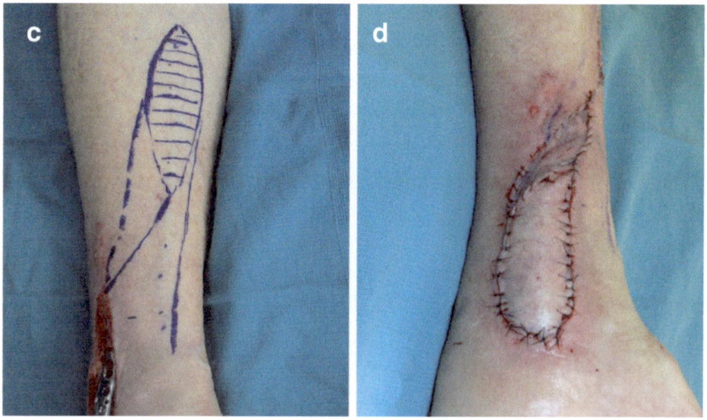

Figure 14.3 (continued)

Venous drainage is primarily via the lesser saphenous vein, which typically has multiple valves preventing retrograde flow. Accompanying collateral veins allow bypass of these valves and facilitate effective outflow [3]. As each contributes to the vascularity of the flap, the median superficial sural artery, lesser saphenous vein, and sural nerve should be included in the flap. Skin paddles as large as 14 cm can be elevated, with a fascial pedicle extending to the pivot point posterosuperior to the lateral malleolus. Fashioning the pivot point at least 5 cm proximal to the lateral malleolus ensures preservation of the distal-most peroneal artery perforators [3].

A reverse sural flap may be reasonable for a defect of moderate size in a patient who is a poor candidate for a free flap, or in facilities not equipped for microsurgery, but it has a well-described complication profile. The retrograde design predisposes it to high rates of congestion and partial flap loss; it should be used cautiously in older patients with diabetes, in those with peripheral vascular disease, or in smokers [3]. Peroneal artery injury or occlusion limits the utility of this flap, and it may be unreliable in patients with posterior tibial artery injury. A “delay” procedure may be necessary to increase the chances of success in co-morbid populations [3].

Pedicled perforator flaps (PPFs) are fasciocutaneous or adipocutaneous flaps based on identified locoregional perforators. They can be based on perforators from any of the major vessels of the distal lower extremity, most commonly the posterior tibial, anterior tibial, or peroneal arteries. In the majority of cases, handheld Doppler can be used preoperatively to identify candidate perforators near the defect, although preoperative vascular imaging is indicated in cases of extensive trauma or in patients with peripheral vascular disease [5]. Flap design is dictated by the reconstructive requirement, and typically takes the form of a rotational flap (like a propeller flap), although advancement designs are also possible. Typically, an island of skin is isolated on a single perforator, which is fully dissected to its source vessel to facilitate flap transposition. The keystone flap similarly relies on fasciocutaneous or musculocutaneous perforators, but it has one key difference: The included perforators may be identified via Doppler, but they are never surgically exposed [6].

The propeller flap is a PPF that relies on rotation as its primary axis of movement. Its oblong shape and rotation about a pivot point resemble those of a propeller. It should be oriented longitudinally to mirror the directionality of vascular flow in the distal lower extremity, with the nourishing vessel placed eccentrically, closer to the defect [6]. The flap is islandized and rotated up to 180° to allow the longer end to resurface the defect. PPFs offer the benefits of reduced operating room times, ideal color and texture match of adjacent tissue, sparing of local muscle, and complication rates similar to those of free flaps [7]. Nevertheless, they can be technically challenging and are not without risks. Kinking of the pedicle (particularly the vein) during rotation can lead to congestion and partial flap loss, with the latter being the most common complication [5, 7]. Advanced patient age (>60 years), diabetes mellitus, and arteriopathy have been identified as risk factors for higher complications [5].

The keystone flap is a multi-perforator advancement flap that can be used to resurface elliptical defects. The trapezoidal shape and flanking V-Y closures lend it mobility, effectively lengthening its short axis as it is advanced towards the defect [6]. Like the propeller flap, the keystone flap is islandized by circumferential incision through the deep fascia, but there is no surgical exposure of the underlying perforators, conferring a distinct advantage by improving technical ease and reducing operating times [8]. Orienting the keystone design longitudinally and on the side of the defect with greater laxity will optimize perfusion and avoid the need to for a secondary skin graft of the donor site. If executed correctly, the keystone flap has a high rate of success. Nonetheless, as with most local options for the lower extremity, partial flap loss is among its complications; it should be used cautiously in co-morbid populations, particularly active smokers [8].

Free Tissue Transfer

The classic approach to distal third reconstruction is free tissue transfer, particularly for defects with a large zone of injury that compromises the integrity and reliability of surrounding tissues. Of primary importance when considering free tissue transfer is the evaluation of vascular inflow to the target anastomotic arteries, which in the distal third are typically the anterior or posterior tibial arteries. Evaluation includes a thorough pulse exam, with arteriography or CT angiography in cases of abnormal exams or if extensive injury questions the vascular integrity. If possible, the reconstructive surgeon should be present for all débridements to ensure that potential recipient vessels are preserved. Vein grafts or arteriovenous loops may be required if the length of the pedicle limits reach outside the zone of injury, which may be the case in some high-energy traumas. Although successful placement of microvascular anastomoses within or distal to the zone of injury has been reported, it should not be considered a first-line option [9, 10].

Of equal importance to recipient vessel evaluation is proper flap selection, which should be guided by the goal of preserving local form and function while minimizing donor site morbidity. In the distal third of the lower extremity, the flap selected should not impede the wearing of clothing or shoes or restrict ankle mobility, which could make ambulation difficult. This can be a delicate balance, as the surgeon should strive to provide robust coverage and effective elimination of dead space without leaving the patient with a bulky lower leg incapable of accommodating a shoe. Whereas the specific flap options are myriad (and often a matter of surgeon preference), certain factors may favor particular options. Important considerations include the volume of the defect, the required pedicle length, and potential donor site morbidity.

Muscle and fasciocutaneous flaps are both reasonable options in extremity reconstruction, as both have demonstrated equivalent limb salvage outcomes [11]. Muscle may be superior in contouring to complex, three-dimensional defects, but the sacrifice of donor muscle (though generally well tolerated) and the appearance of skin-grafted muscle are among its disadvantages. The latissimus dorsi flap is an excellent option for large, even circumferential defects of the distal leg. The rectus abdominis flap can also provide coverage of larger defects, but it has fallen out of favor in recent years owing to the resultant abdominal wall weakness and potential abdominal bulging. Regardless, both offer robust, pliable muscle with a pedicle of sufficient length and caliber, and can usually allow reach beyond the zone of injury. The gracilis flap is yet another option, and is an excellent choice for smaller defects. It offers an excellent donor site profile, with little to no functional loss and a scar well hidden in the medial thigh [1].

In recent decades, improved understanding of vascular perforasomes has led to a rise in the use of fasciocutaneous perforator flaps for lower extremity reconstruction [1]. These allow for muscle preservation, which means no risk of functional loss, but the tradeoff is often a less aesthetic donor site that may need grafting. Fasciocutaneous perforator flaps may be preferred in situations where re-elevation is anticipated for future bone grafting or definitive fixation of concomitant fractures [11]. Among the many options, the anterolateral thigh (ALT) flap is often considered the workhorse flap in lower extremity reconstruction [4]. It is highly versatile and can be elevated as a chimeric flap based off the lateral circumflex system, with inclusion of the vastus lateralis or portions of the tensor fascia lata if additional bulk is needed (Fig. 14.4). However, even without muscle, it may prove too bulky for superficial defects, especially in obese patients with significant subcutaneous tissue at the thigh. Though secondary de-bulking is an option, a thinner flap may be may be more apt. The radial forearm flap is sufficiently thin, and lends itself well to the "skin only" area of the anterior shin. Like the ALT, it has a long vascular pedicle, although the placement of the donor site over the highly visible volar forearm may be unacceptable

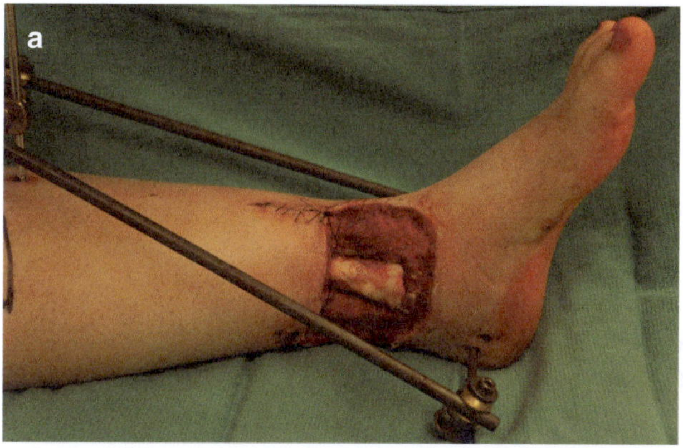

Figure 14.4 Free anterolateral thigh (ALT) flap. This patient suffered a composite bone and soft tissue defect of the left ankle after a fall from height. (**a**) After serial débridement, an antibiotic spacer was placed in the bone defect and lower leg stability and length were maintained with an external fixator. (**b**) A large ALT flap was designed on the contralateral thigh. The flap was designed with excess size greater than the defect in order to provide durable soft tissue bulk and coverage of the posterior tibial artery vascular pedicle. (**c**) This also ensures sufficient soft tissue coverage for the flap to be elevated subsequently for bone grafting and internal hardware placement. Note the posterior extension of the external fixator to provide elevation of the lower leg and ankle, to avoid pressure on the vascular anastomosis

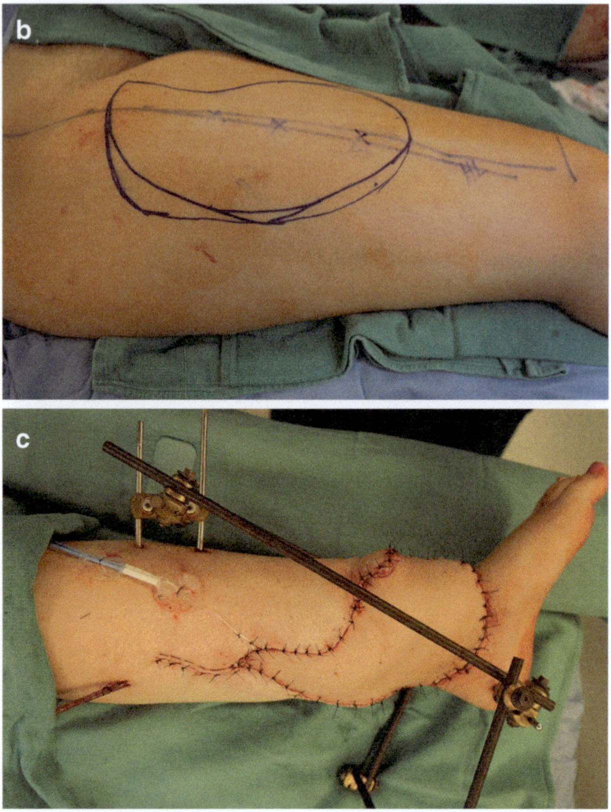

Figure 14.4 (continued)

to some patients. Other options worthy of mention include the lateral arm and parascapular flaps, as well as the perforator variants of the aforementioned muscular flaps—the thoracodorsal artery perforator and deep inferior epigastric artery perforator flaps. Although reliable, these see much less use than the previously described fasciocutaneous flaps.

Postoperative Care

Most free flap failures occur within the first 24 hours after surgery, so care should be taken to closely monitor flap viability in this time [1]. Local and regional flaps should be monitored for congestion or areas of tissue compromise. Postoperative elevation of the extremity can reduce the chance of venous congestion and facilitate vascular accommodation of the flap.

Physiotherapy and gait retraining are vital in the postoperative recovery, and are introduced gradually, although weight-bearing status is dependent on the involvement of bony structures in the initial defect. A multidisciplinary approach to postoperative recovery is best, involving input from reconstructive surgeons, orthopaedic surgeons, and physical and occupational therapists. In some cases, secondary revision procedures may be performed for flap debulking or scar release for functional and aesthetic concerns.

Summary

Free tissue transfer is the primary modality of soft tissue reconstruction for the distal third of the lower extremity, although regional flaps (which obviate the need for microsurgical anastomoses) may be viable options in select cases. Larger defects or those with significant local inflammation or zone of injury are best reconstructed with a free flap, as long as the patient's general health status will allow it. Thorough assessment of the vascular status of the extremity is critical, and further imaging should be used on a case-by-case basis. Postoperative care and rehabilitation are crucial elements to a good, functional reconstruction.

References

1. Soltanian H, Garcia RM, Hollenbeck ST. Current concepts in lower extremity reconstruction. Plast Reconstr Surg. 2015;136:815e–29e.
2. Granzow JW, Li A, Suliman A, Caton A, Goldberg M, Boyd JB. Bipedicled flaps in posttraumatic lower-extremity reconstruction. J Plast Reconstr Aesthet Surg. 2013;66:1415–20.
3. Follmar KE, Baccarani A, Baumeister SP, Levin LS, Erdmann D. The distally based sural flap. Plast Reconstr Surg. 2007;119:138e–48e.
4. Lachica RD. Evidence-based medicine: management of acute lower extremity trauma. Plast Reconstr Surg. 2017;139:287e–301e.
5. Bekara F, Herlin C, Mojallal A, Sinna R, Ayestaray B, Letois F, et al. A systematic review and meta-analysis of perforator-pedicled propeller flaps in lower extremity defects: identification of risk factors for complications. Plast Reconstr Surg. 2016;137:314–31.
6. Abraham JT, Saint-Cyr M. Keystone and pedicle perforator flaps in reconstructive surgery: new modifications and applications. Clin Plast Surg. 2017;44:385–402.
7. Bekara F, Herlin C, Somda S, de Runz A, Grolleau JL, Chaput B. Free versus perforator-pedicled propeller flaps in lower extremity reconstruction: what is the safest coverage? A meta-analysis. Microsurgery. 2018;38:109–19.
8. Khouri JS, Egeland BM, Daily SD, Harake MS, Kwon S, Neligan PC, et al. The keystone island flap: use in large defects of the trunk and extremities in soft-tissue reconstruction. Plast Reconstr Surg. 2011;127:1212–21.
9. Spector JA, Levine S, Levine JP. Free tissue transfer to the lower extremity distal to the zone of injury: indications and outcomes over a 25-year experience. Plast Reconstr Surg. 2007;120:952–9.
10. Bendon CL, Giele HP. Success of free flap anastomoses performed within the zone of trauma in acute lower limb reconstruction. J Plast Reconstr Aesthet Surg. 2016;69:888–93.
11. Cho EH, Shammas RL, Carney MJ, Weissler JM, Bauder AR, Glener AD, et al. Muscle versus fasciocutaneous free flaps in lower extremity traumatic reconstruction: a multicenter outcomes analysis. Plast Reconstr Surg. 2018;141:191–9.

Chapter 15
Soft Tissue Reconstruction of the Foot

Whitney O. Lane, Ronnie L. Shammas, and Scott T. Hollenbeck

The primary goal in foot reconstruction after trauma is to preserve function of the entire lower limb by helping to restore a stable weight-bearing surface that allows for painless ambulation. Additional considerations include ease of shoe fitting and aesthetic form of the reconstructed foot. When foot reconstruction is not possible or is complicated by failure or infection, the patient is at risk for undergoing a below-knee amputation.

W. O. Lane
Division of Plastic, Maxillofacial, and Oral Surgery, Duke University Medical Center, Durham, NC, USA

R. L. Shammas
Division of Plastic, Maxillofacial, and Oral Surgery, Duke University Health System, Durham, NC, USA

S. T. Hollenbeck (✉)
Division of Plastic and Reconstructive Surgery, Duke University Medical Center, Durham, NC, USA
e-mail: scott.hollenbeck@duke.edu

S. T. Hollenbeck et al. (eds.), *Handbook of Lower Extremity Reconstruction*, https://doi.org/10.1007/978-3-030-41035-3_15

Foot Anatomy and Function

The foot can be considered in terms of forefoot, midfoot, and heel. Each area has its own functional demands. Similarly, the dorsum of the foot has very thin, mobile skin, whereas the plantar aspect has thick, adherent, glabrous skin and underlying plantar aponeurosis. Stable underlying bony architecture is required for efficient and pain-free ambulation.

The main vascular supply to the foot comes from the posterior tibial artery (Fig. 15.1). The artery splits into the medial and lateral plantar arteries beneath the flexor retinaculum within the tarsal tunnel. These two arteries join at the base of the metatarsals to form the deep plantar arch. The lateral plantar artery is the dominant artery supplying the fourth and fifth toes through metatarsal and then proper digital arteries. The medial artery supplies the first through third toes in a similar fashion. The dorsalis pedis artery supplies the dorsum of the foot and also gives terminal branches completing the plantar arch. For reconstructive purposes, the plantar intrinsic muscles of the foot are typically supplied via the medial and lateral plantar arteries.

Cutaneous sensation to the forefoot is supplied via terminal branches of the sciatic nerve. Sensation on the plantar surface of the forefoot is mainly derived from the medial plantar nerve (tibial origin) and the lateral plantar nerves (tibial origin). The dorsal forefoot sensation is mainly derived from the superficial peroneal nerves (common peroneal origin) and the unique first web space distribution of the deep peroneal nerve (common peroneal, sciatic, L5 origin). Motor innervation of the intrinsic foot muscles is mainly through the medial and lateral plantar nerves.

Free Flaps Versus Local Flaps

Local flap options for the foot are well established [1, 2]. However, local flaps are typically limited by the small size of the muscles and a limited arc of rotation. Regional flaps for the foot are typically fasciocutaneous flaps and rely on perforators or reverse flow [3]. Muscles in the leg typically have proximal blood supply and do not lend themselves to rotation to the foot. For

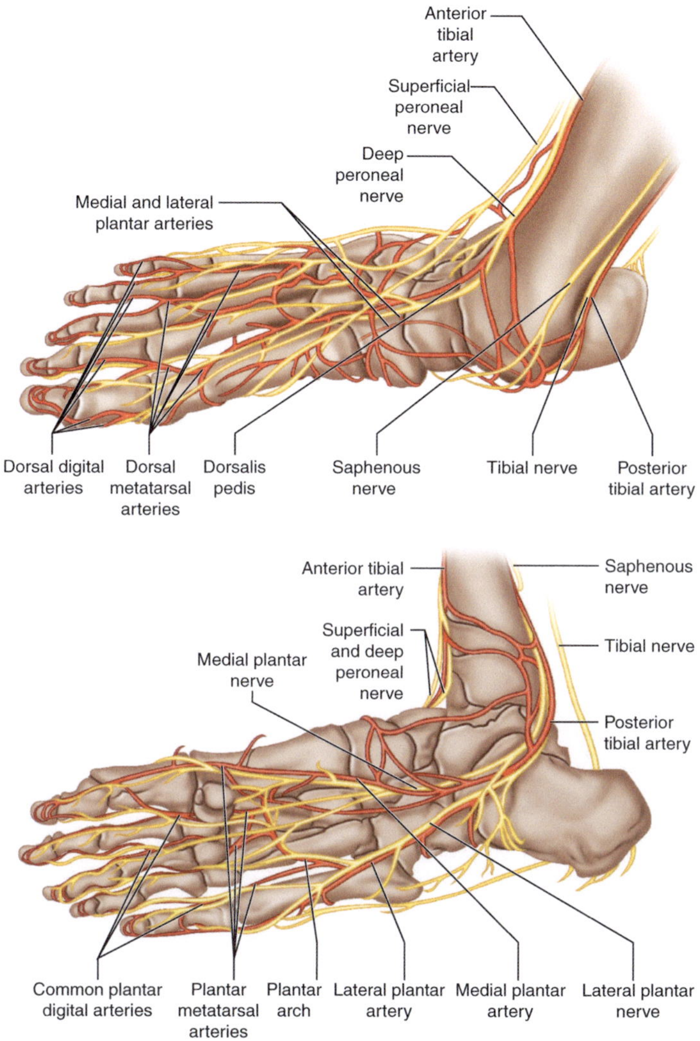

Figure 15.1 Anatomy of the foot and ankle with artery and nerves

larger defects, free tissue transfer is typically a reliable method for reconstruction [4]. Free flap options are dictated by surgeon expertise and the size and location of the defect, in the context of the subunit principle illustrated in Fig. 15.2 and Table 15.1 [5].

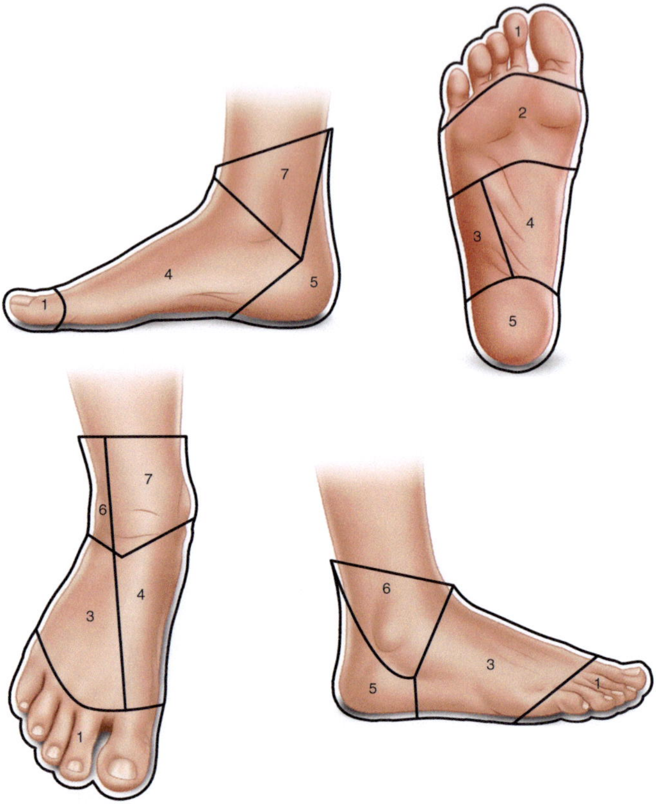

Subunit	Demands: Tissue Needs	Optimal Flaps
1	Low functional, Moderate aesthetic: small, thin and pliable.	Radial forearm > lateral arm
2	High functional, Low aesthetic: durable and minimal bulk.	(*): Radial forearm > lateral arm > gracilis with STSG > ALT
3/4	Low functional, High aesthetic: smooth, thin and pliable.	Radial forearm > ALT > scapular > latissimus dorsi
5	High functional, Low aesthetic: durable and moderate bulk.	(*): ALT> gracilis with STSG > latissimus dorsi > scapular > lateral arm > radial forearm
6/7	Moderate functional, Moderate aesthetic; may vary from smooth, thin and pliable to large and bulky.	Gracilis with STSG, latissimus dorsi, ALT, rectus abdominis, lateral arm, radial forearm, scapular

STSG: Split thickness skin graft
ALT: Anterolateral thigh
*: Nerve coaptation may be considered

FIGURE 15.2 Subunits of the foot for flap reconstruction, which can be used as a guideline for choosing flaps to cover defects of the foot and ankle, as listed in Table 15.1

TABLE 15.1 *Choice of free flap options* for reconstruction of subunits of the foot

Subunit	Demands	Tissue needs	Optimal flaps
1	Low functional, moderate aesthetic	Small, thin, and pliable	Radial forearm > lateral arm
2	High functional, low aesthetic	Durable, with minimal bulk	(∗) Radial forearm > lateral arm > gracilis with STSG > ALT
3/4	Low functional, high aesthetic	Smooth, thin, and pliable	Radial forearm > ALT > scapular> latissimus dorsi
5	High functional, low aesthetic	Durable, with moderate bulk	(∗) ALT > gracilis with STSG > latissimus dorsi > scapular > lateral arm > radial forearm
6/7	Moderate functional, moderate aesthetic	May vary from smooth, thin, and pliable to large and bulky	Gracilis with STSG, latissimus dorsi, ALT, rectus abdominis, lateral arm, radial forearm, scapular

ALT anterolateral thigh, *STSG* split-thickness skin graft
[a]Nerve coaptation may be considered

Local and Regional Flaps for the Heel

Defects involving the heel may be simple or complex, depending on involvement of the calcaneus and Achilles tendon. Additionally, trauma-related wounds often are accompanied by substantial local injury that precludes local and regional flaps. For simple defects that involve loss of skin over the calcaneus, local and regional flaps may be used. The reverse sural fasciocutaneous or adipocutaneous flap is a regional flap based on retrograde flow from perforators of the peroneal and posterior tibial artery as well as the vasa nervorum of the sural nerve. The flap has a high rate of complications related to poor circulation [6], but the "delay technique" (Fig. 15.3) may be used to improve outcomes [7].

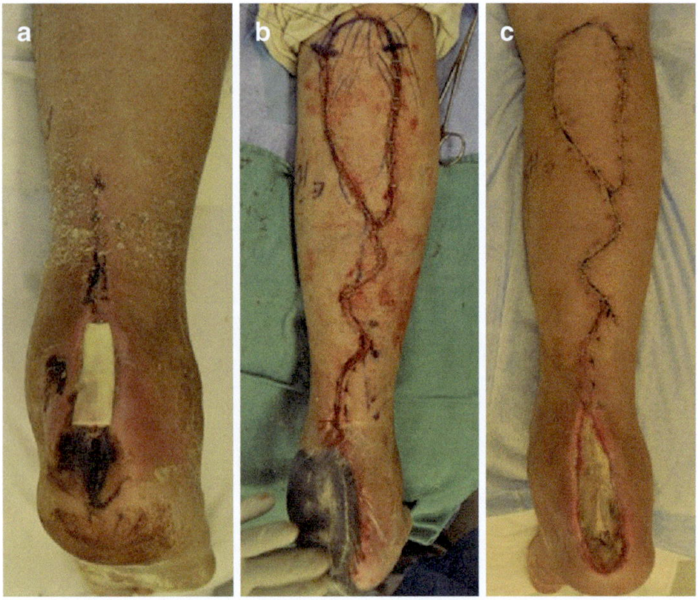

FIGURE 15.3 Reverse sural flap for Achilles coverage. (**a**) This patient had necrotic skin and breakdown following a posterior approach for ankle fusion. (**b**) Initially, the reverse sural flap is created using vascular and skin delay principles. The proximal portion of the skin is kept intact to act as a nutrient source for the skin island. The wound is débrided and negative pressure therapy is applied. (**c**) After waiting 2 weeks, the wound and the reverse sural flap both appear healthy. The proximal skin bridge has been divided in the outpatient setting. (**d**) The reverse sural flap has been rotated into position. A skin graft has been used to cover the donor defect and a portion of the pedicle. (**e**) The flap is shown to be healed in place 3 months after surgery. (*Photos courtesy of* Scott T. Hollenbeck, MD)

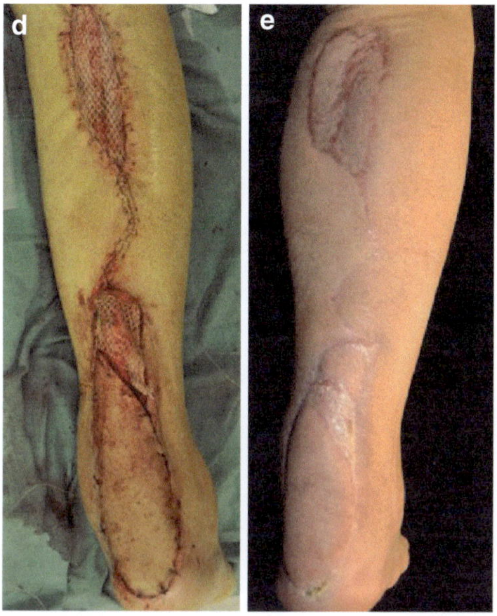

FIGURE 15.3 (continued)

Perforator flaps from the distal leg can be used to reach the heel region (Fig. 15.4). These flaps are often small and necessitate significant rotation, which can compromise blood flow in the short perforator pedicle. Thus, extensive edema and local inflammation preclude use of these flaps.

Local flaps from within the foot can be used to cover heel defects. The medial plantar or "instep" flap (Fig. 15.5) has the advantage that it may be sensate and provide plantar-based skin for resurfacing the heel [1]. The donor defect requires a skin graft but is on a non–weight-bearing surface. This flap is also limited to situations in which local edema and trauma are minimal.

Local muscle flaps may also be used for covering heel defects. These include the flexor digitorum brevis (FDB) flap, the abductor digiti minimi (ADM) flap, and the abductor hallucis (AH) flap. These flaps are small and useful only for certain defects.

Free Flaps for the Heel

Complex defects involving the heel often include injury to the calcaneus and the Achilles tendon and are associated with significant local injury [8]. In these cases, free tissue transfer is needed. Muscle flaps (such as the gracilis) or fasciocutaneous flaps (such as the ALT) can provide stable weight-bearing coverage for the heel (Fig. 15.6) [4]. The Achilles tendon can be reconstructed with allograft or autograft. The fascia lata

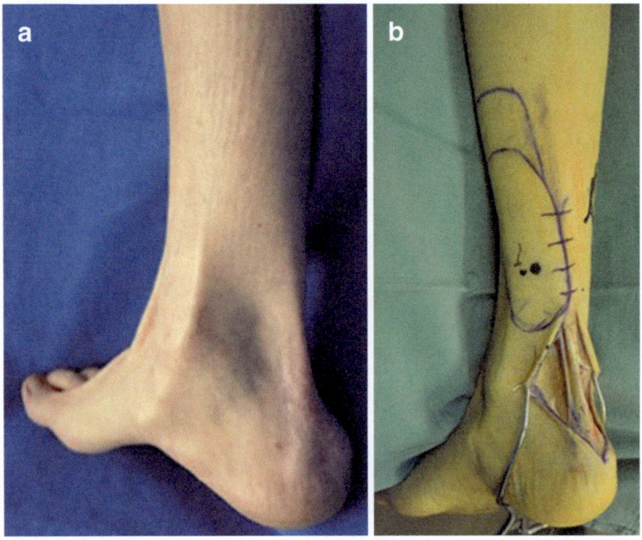

FIGURE 15.4 Perforator flap for heel wound. (**a**) This patient had a partially ruptured Achilles tendon and thin, attenuated skin overlying the tendon. (**b**) A perforator flap is designed based on the posterior tibial artery and a skin perforator. The *dot* indicates the Doppler signal from the perforator. The underlying tendon repair is performed. (**c**) The flap has been elevated and rotated into position. Given the short length of the perforator, the flap has been only partially rotated at the proximal portion. (**d**) The flap appears viable and shows good interface healing at 2 weeks after surgery. A skin graft has been used for the donor defect. (*Photos courtesy of* Scott T. Hollenbeck, MD)

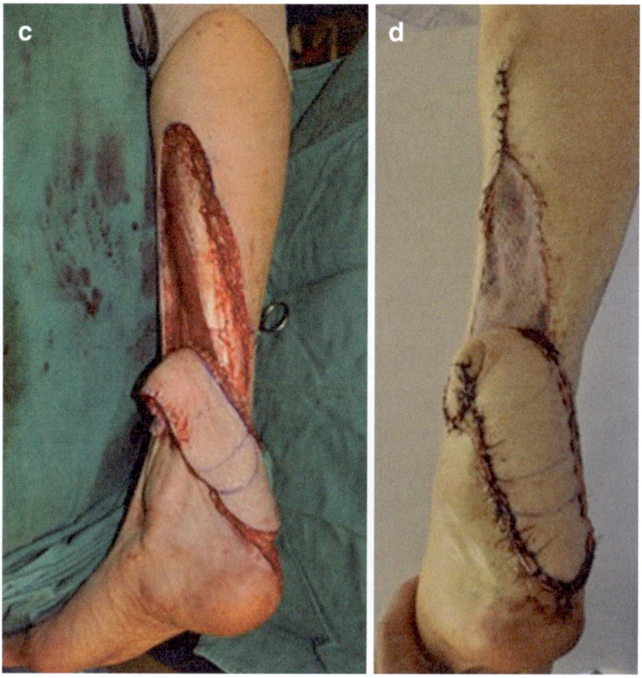

FIGURE 15.4 (continued)

is an excellent source of tissue for this purpose. Recipient vessels for heel reconstruction typically are the posterior tibial artery and vein [9]. The saphenous vein can be used as a recipient vein, but it may be thickened because of inflammation and edema.

Flaps for the Dorsal Foot

The skin of the dorsal foot is extremely thin. Following an injury or wound, the underlying tendons and bone are susceptible to injury and dissection. Soft tissue coverage of the dorsal foot typically is performed with free tissue transfer.

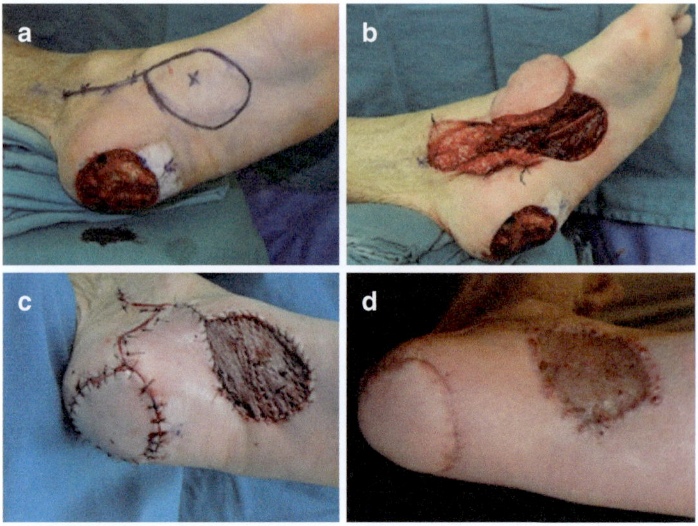

FIGURE 15.5 Heel defect coverage with medial plantar flap. (**a**) A localized heel defect following cancer removal: A medial plantar flap is designed. (**b**) The flap has been elevated on the medial plantar vessel. A branch of the medial plantar nerve can be maintained to provide flap sensation. (**c**) The flap has been rotated into position and a skin graft has been placed on the donor defect. (**d**) The flap is shown 6 weeks after surgery, with good interface healing. (*Photos courtesy of* Detlev Erdmann, MD)

Flaps used for this purpose need to be thin and have vessels that will match well with the dorsalis pedis. The radial forearm flap (Fig. 15.7) and the superficial circumflex iliac artery perforator flap are often used for this purpose [10].

Postoperative Care

Foot reconstruction is often associated with long periods of leg elevation and non–weight-bearing status. When the wounds and fractures have healed, the patient may begin to walk in a boot or other form of support. Long-term care centers on stability of the reconstruction over time. Large,

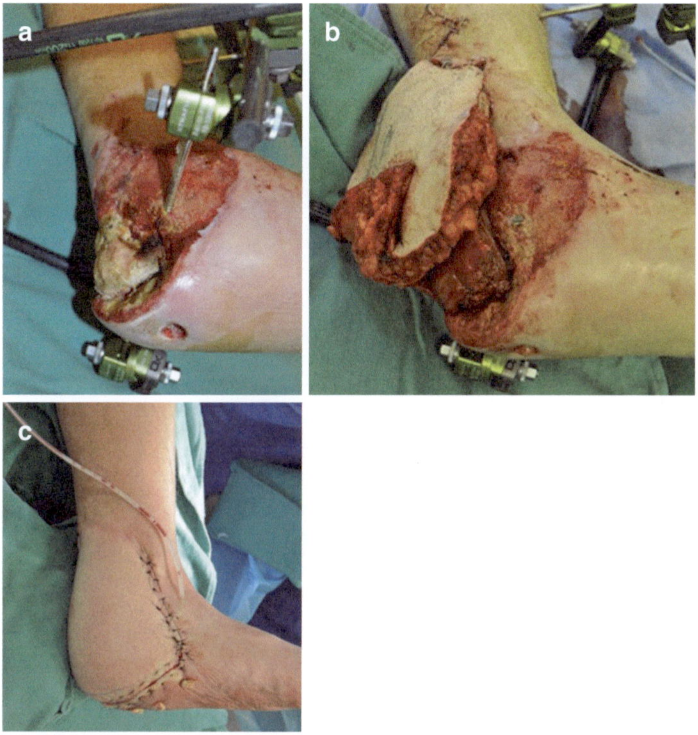

FIGURE 15.6 Traumatic defect of the heel. (**a**) This large and complex defect of the heel included fracture and exposure of the calcaneus bone. (**b**) A free flap (anterolateral thigh [ALT] with vastus lateralis muscle) has been created and delivered to the heel region. The muscle has been placed directly over the fracture and exposed bone. (**c**) At 6 months, the flap was well healed and amenable to a flap-debulking procedure. The final result after debulking is shown. (*Photos courtesy of* Scott T. Hollenbeck, MD)

bulky flaps often require debulking procedures to improve shoe fitting. Plantar flaps are prone to breakdown and must be followed. Shoe inserts may help defer weight off the flap, and orthotics may even be necessary to improve gait. Finally, bony prominences may need to be taken down if there are signs of excess pressure on the flap.

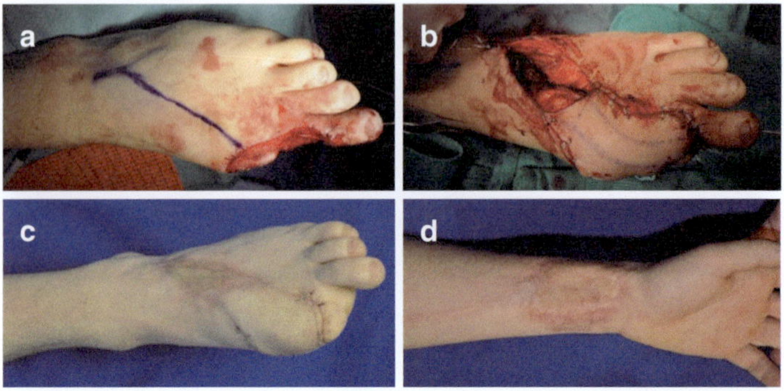

FIGURE 15.7 Radial forearm free flap for dorsal foot wound. (**a**) Amputation of the first toe resulted in a complex wound of the distal foot. (**b**) A radial forearm free flap has been used to cover the defect. (**c**) Six months following surgery, the flap is well healed and provides stable soft tissue coverage. (**d**) The donor defect has been closed with a skin graft, which shows excellent healing. (*Photos courtesy of* Scott T. Hollenbeck, MD)

Summary

Foot reconstruction can be extremely challenging because of the unique skin in this area, the distal blood flow, high functional demand, and the lack of available local options. Complex foot wounds may result from trauma. Failure of the reconstruction in either skin stability or bony non-union is often associated with below-knee amputation. Careful planning and extensive postoperative care are needed to achieve limb salvage. Less complex wounds can be managed with a variety of techniques and are associated with good functional outcomes.

References

1. Yang D, Yang JF, Morris SF, Tang M, Nie C. Medial plantar artery perforator flap for soft-tissue reconstruction of the heel. Ann Plast Surg. 2011;67:294–8.

2. Ducic I, Attinger CE. Foot and ankle reconstruction: pedicled muscle flaps versus free flaps and the role of diabetes. Plast Reconstr Surg. 2011;128:173–80.
3. Parrett BM, Pribaz JJ, Matros E, Przylecki W, Sampson CE, Orgill DP. Risk analysis for the reverse sural fasciocutaneous flap in distal leg reconstruction. Plast Reconstr Surg. 2009;123:1499–504.
4. Zhu YL, Wang Y, He XQ, Zhu M, Li FB, Xu YQ. Foot and ankle reconstruction: an experience on the use of 14 different flaps in 226 cases. Microsurgery. 2013;33:600–4.
5. Hollenbeck ST, Woo S, Komatsu I, Erdmann D, Zenn MR, Levin LS. Longitudinal outcomes and application of the subunit principle to 165 foot and ankle free tissue transfers. Plast Reconstr Surg. 2010;125:924–34.
6. Baumeister SP, Spierer R, Erdmann D, Sweis R, Levin LS, Germann GK. A realistic complication analysis of 70 sural artery flaps in a multimorbid patient group. Plast Reconstr Surg. 2003;112:129–40; discussion 141–2.
7. Erdmann D, Levin S. Delayed reverse sural flap for staged reconstruction of the foot and lower leg. Plast Reconstr Surg. 2006;118:571–2.
8. Cho EH, Garcia R, Pien I, Thomas S, Levin LS, Hollenbeck ST. An algorithmic approach for managing orthopaedic surgical wounds of the foot and ankle. Clin Orthop Relat Res. 2014;472:1921–9.
9. Cho EH, Garcia RM, Pien I, Kuchibhatla M, Levinson H, Erdmann D, et al. Vascular considerations in foot and ankle free tissue transfer: analysis of 231 free flaps. Microsurgery. 2016;36:276–83.
10. Hong JP, Sun SH, Ben-Nakhi M. Modified superficial circumflex iliac artery perforator flap and supermicrosurgery technique for lower extremity reconstruction: a new approach for moderate-sized defects. Ann Plast Surg. 2013;71:380–3.

Chapter 16
Amputation Principles and Targeted Muscle Reinnervation

Sean Figy, Ryan C. Jefferson, and Ian L. Valerio

Fundamentals of Amputation

Amputation of an extremity is a common procedure performed for a variety of indications. For lower extremity amputations, certain co-morbid states (peripheral vascular disease, diabetes, etc.), trauma, oncology, and congenital deformities all contribute patients who may require amputation for medical or functional needs. Amputation can be

S. Figy
Department of Surgery, The University of Nebraska Medical Center, Omaha, NE, USA

R. C. Jefferson
Department of Plastic and Reconstructive Surgery, The Ohio State University Wexner Medical Center, Columbus, OH, USA

I. L. Valerio (✉)
Division of Burn, Wound, and Trauma, Departments of Plastic & Reconstructive, General, and Orthopaedic Surgery, The Ohio State University Wexner Medical Center, Columbus, OH, USA
e-mail: ian.valerio@osumc.edu

S. T. Hollenbeck et al. (eds.), *Handbook of Lower Extremity Reconstruction*, https://doi.org/10.1007/978-3-030-41035-3_16

performed at varying levels based on the patient's need, including partial foot amputation, below-knee or above-knee amputation, or hip disarticulation. Regardless of the reason and site of amputation, there are a set of common principles of amputation that can aid in achieving the best functional outcome for the residual limb [1]. Figure 16.1 summarizes the most common levels of amputation and the most common associated motor nerve targets at each level.

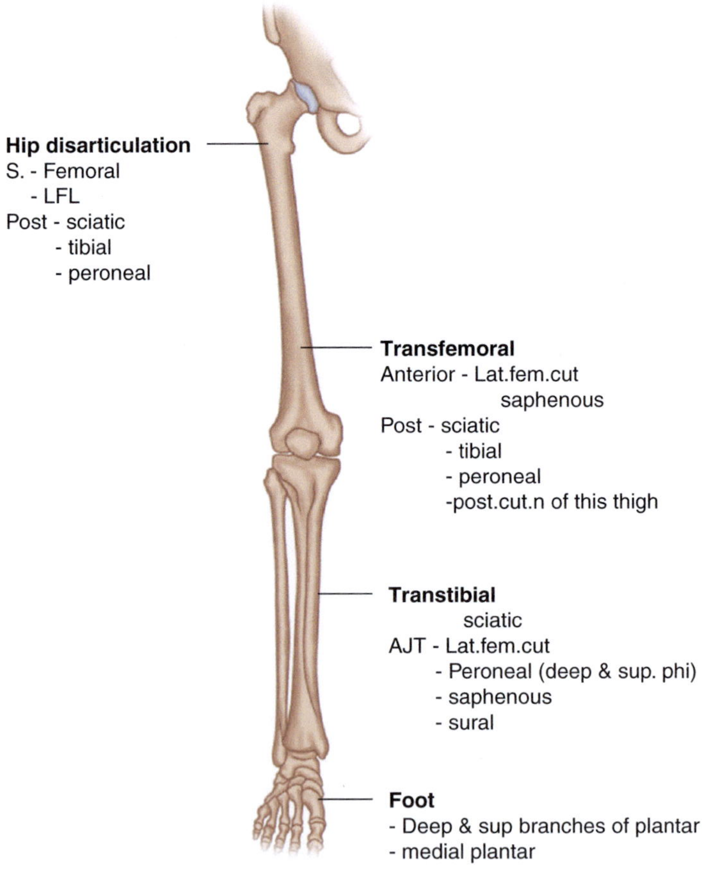

Figure 16.1 Amputation levels, presented with the different nerve targets for each level

Level of Amputation

Lower extremity amputation can include a number of sites:

- Hip disarticulation
- Transfemoral or above-knee amputation (AKA)
- Knee disarticulation or through-knee amputation (TKA)
- Transtibial or below-knee amputation (BKA)
- Amputations of the foot, either partial or complete

In general, it is preferred to keep the maximal residual limb length for purposes of minimizing energy expenditure and maximizing native function. The added benefits of preserving maximal length have been well documented and are generally known [2]. Table 16.1 details the increased energy expenditure with ambulation associated with different levels of amputation.

In addition to a reduced energy requirement with prosthetic wear and use, more distal amputation levels are also generally associated with better functionality. The more proximal an amputation is, the more an amputee patient must accommodate for the increased number of lost joints. Preservation of more distal joints increases functionality by maintaining more degrees of natural movement [3].

Though this is a relatively intuitive and simple concept, it can become more challenging to choose an appropriate level of amputation in certain patient populations, in which other considerations arise (Table 16.2). Patient circumstances sometimes may favor a more proximal amputation; the deci-

Table 16.1 Increased energy requirements by amputation site

Level of amputation	Energy expenditure above baseline
Transtibial (unilateral)	120–125%
Transtibial (bilateral)	140%
Transfemoral (unilateral)	160–170%
Transfemoral (bilateral)	>200%

From Meier and Melton [3]; with permission

Table 16.2 Considerations for determination of amputation level

Consideration	Determining factors
Patient goals	Patients may have a preferred level of amputation
Functional status	It is important to consider the patient's baseline functional status when choosing appropriate amputation technique
Contralateral extremity	Many patients have a contralateral amputation, which may change decision-making about the ipsilateral site
Oncology	Safe oncologic margins may sometimes abut preferred levels of amputation. In these circumstances, it may be chosen to alter the level of amputation to maximize quality of resection
Medical comorbidities	The patient may not be medically or physically capable to heal, rehabilitate, or use a prosthetic
Soft tissue quality	Absence of healthy soft tissue may necessitate a more proximal amputation
Available prostheses	The availability of certain prosthetics and the teams to implement them may be limited for certain populations

sion may be based on conversations with the patient and the expertise of the surgical, rehabilitation, and prosthetic teams.

Soft Tissue Management

Although amputation is typically thought of in terms of bone length, the soft tissue is a critical consideration for function and the success of prosthetic wear. Failure to adequately manage the residual soft tissues can result in a multitude of complications such as chronic wounds, soft tissue erosion or ulceration (with potential for bone infection), failure of prosthetic tolerance, and discomfort or pain. The key to soft tissue management in amputation is finding an acceptable soft tissue equilibrium and balance for maximal prosthetic function. A number of techniques have been found to be successful in optimizing soft tissue coverage:

- Leaving adequate soft tissue to maximize wound healing potential and padding of pressure points without leaving excess bulk, which can contribute to poor prosthetic fit. Carving the bone edges to remove sharp pressure points further helps prevent breakdown.
- Optimize scar placement to minimize tension, shearing, and discomfort, while maximizing cosmesis and wound healing.
- Balance the actions of the residual musculature to align the residual limb into a functional position. This is accomplished through thoughtful, technically sound myodesis, attaching the residual musculature to the bony stump. This is especially critical when addressing the adductor/abductor system of the thigh in transfemoral amputation [4].
- Leave local musculature attached to periosteum to optimize control of future prostheses.
- Tailor the shape of the muscular envelope and soft tissues to snugly fit into a prosthetic while still avoiding pressure on the bony stump. Using a cruciform drill technique (in which drill holes are placed 1 cm proximal to the cut end of the bone in the transverse and anterior-posterior dimensions), a transosseus myodesis helps balance and further pad the remaining bony stump.
- Address neurovascular bundles thoughtfully. Meticulous hemostasis of major vessels is critical to avoid hematoma. Traction neurectomy was previously used to treat the residual major peripheral nerves, but advanced techniques such as targeted muscle reinnervation (TMR) provide refinements in amputation that have been shown to reduce painful or symptomatic neuroma development as well as phantom limb and residual limb pain; they also optimize the potential for the use of biointegrated or neuromodulated bioprosthetics.

These points are even more important in the care of patients undergoing revision amputation with conversion to a higher level or modifications to existing residual limbs.

Multidisciplinary Care

Though an amputation is a surgical procedure, it is of the utmost importance to employ a multidisciplinary approach. Limb transplantation has been described is not a common event and is unlikely to become the standard of care for most patients suffering from lower limb loss. Thus, lower limb amputation is permanent and will have lifelong implications, so it is important to work in conjunction with multiple disciplines to give the patient the best outcome possible. When available, the team approach to amputation should include a medical specialist, who can optimize the patient for surgery and manage comorbidities such as diabetes and peripheral vascular disease. The surgical team should consist of the amputation surgeon specialist (most often orthopaedic, vascular, plastic, and/or general surgery) and a plastic surgeon to address the remaining soft tissues and provide peripheral nerve treatment advances, including TMR. Lastly, the rehabilitation specialists should be involved (ideally preoperatively, to connect the patient with the necessary education and amputee support groups). The role of rehabilitation for the amputee cannot be overstated. The surgical amputation is truly the beginning of the journey for the patient, who will need lifelong postoperative rehabilitation and prosthetic modification or optimization.

Fundamentals of Targeted Muscle Reinnervation (TMR)

Targeted muscle reinnervation (TMR) was initially developed to allow upper extremity amputees better intuitive control of myoelectric prostheses and bioprostheses by reestablishing some function of the amputated nerve via multiple bioamplifiers. In 2004, Kuiken et al. [5] first described the concept in a patient who underwent brachial plexus nerve transfers to divided regions of the pectoralis muscles, thus creating discrete areas of innervation dubbed "myoneurosomes." These areas had nerve signals detectable on EMG and could subsequently be employed as bioamplifiers for control of a myoelectric prosthesis. The subsequent patients who underwent TMR demonstrated better speed and control of their prosthetics. Recently, an exciting incidental finding, which was further evaluated and proven in multiple later clinical research studies [6, 7] was that TMR patients experienced significant decreases in symptomatic neuroma formation, phantom limb pain (PLP), and residual limb pain (RLP). These benefits were seen as far out as 10 years after TMR [6].

Prior to TMR, treatment of symptomatic neuroma pain was inconsistent and showed varying results. The treatment options were grouped into the categories of pharmacology, psychology, and physical manipulation in the form of therapy or surgery. None of these options, either alone or combined, enjoyed consistent success that could establish a standard of care. In contrast, TMR is a more predictable, consistent, and reproducible technique that has shown success in decreasing symptomatic neuroma and phantom limb pain, with the added benefit of improved control of advanced prosthetics. The fundamental concept of TMR is to perform a nerve transfer of a residual peripheral sensory or mixed motor-sensory nerve to a target motor nerve within the residual muscles of the amputation stump. The target motor nerve is a redundant muscular motor nerve within the field of amputation. This end-to-end nerve transfer and associated coaptation facilitates organized nerve regeneration into the recipient donor motor nerve and motor end plates of the freshly deinnervated target muscle. By restoring physical continuity, the nerve is provided with "somewhere to go and something to do." Reinnervating the denervated target muscles decreases the disorganized nerve regeneration that leads to symptomatic neuroma formation, as well as phantom and residual limb pain.

Technical Pearls of TMR

A number of critical points during TMR are worthy of highlighting to optimize the desired outcomes:

- **Management of existing neuroma in delayed amputation cases.** In general, one should excise the neuroma in its entirety from those major peripheral nerves set to be transferred. Often this neuroma is easily palpable, firm, and able to be dissected from the surrounding tissues. It is important, however, to dissect the nerve proximal enough that healthy nerve tissue and axon levels are achieved, to permit nerve regeneration and growth toward the targeted motor nerve, for the muscle to be reinnervated. An indicator of a healthy nerve level is close observation of endoneurial bleeding after the major peripheral nerve for pending transfer is cut sharply.
- **Careful nerve handling.** Peripheral nerves are delicate structures and must be handled with care to prevent inadvertent axonal injury that could lead to scarring, loss of axon viability, and internal damage that may inhibit nerve regeneration and growth. Once the nerves are encountered during surgical dissection, the use of high-resolution magnification and atraumatic microsurgical instruments is recommended. The use of electrocautery or bipolar electrosurgery should be kept to a minimum to prevent thermal injury to the neural contents.
- **Identification of target nerves.** The identification of target nerves can be challenging. Often the target motor nerve branch is thin and lacks the structural integrity of the major peripheral nerve to which it will be coapted. The use of intraoperative hand-held and on-field nerve stimulators has made the task of identifying target nerves easier and has reduced the operative time associated with TMR surgery.
- **Coaptation.** The coaptation of the major sensory and mixed motor-sensory peripheral nerves to the target motor nerves are the interfaces across which the nerves

will regenerate to reinnervate their target muscles. After the target nerve is identified, it should be transected sharply, to minimize inadvertent injury. These nerves that are embedded in muscle have a propensity to retract, so it is often a safe move to place the first bite of microsuture within the target nerve epineurium before transection, to avoid losing the cut end of the nerve to retraction back into its surrounding muscle. Coaptation should be performed under magnification with appropriate-sized microsuture to maximize accuracy and reduce inadvertent injury and inflammation. Care should be taken to avoid inclusion or strangulation of the fascicles within the sutures, as this can crush the nerve fascicles or contribute to scar formation, which may inhibit nerve regeneration (Fig. 16.2). The coaptation should be performed near the entrance of the motor nerve into the target muscle and should have minimal tension to avoid disruption. If a hand-held nerve stimulator is available, it can be used afterwards to test the integrity of the coaptation. Stimulation of the peripheral nerve should produce a motor response in the target muscle if the nerve transfer was performed well.

- **Soft tissue management.** The success of TMR potentially can be sabotaged by oversights elsewhere in the operation. Once TMR has been performed, it is advised to use the local denervated muscle as a wrap over the coaptation. This serves the function of protecting the nerve repair as well as insulating it from other nerve transfers that may have been performed in the local area. Additional adjunctive nerve coaptation assistive devices, such as nerve wraps or connectors, may also be considered to aid in protecting the nerve coaptations, if desired. Once the nerve transfer has been completed, diligent attention should be paid to the other principles of soft tissue management discussed above. Failure to attentively manage the soft tissues of the amputation can sabotage any gain made by TMR [6, 7].

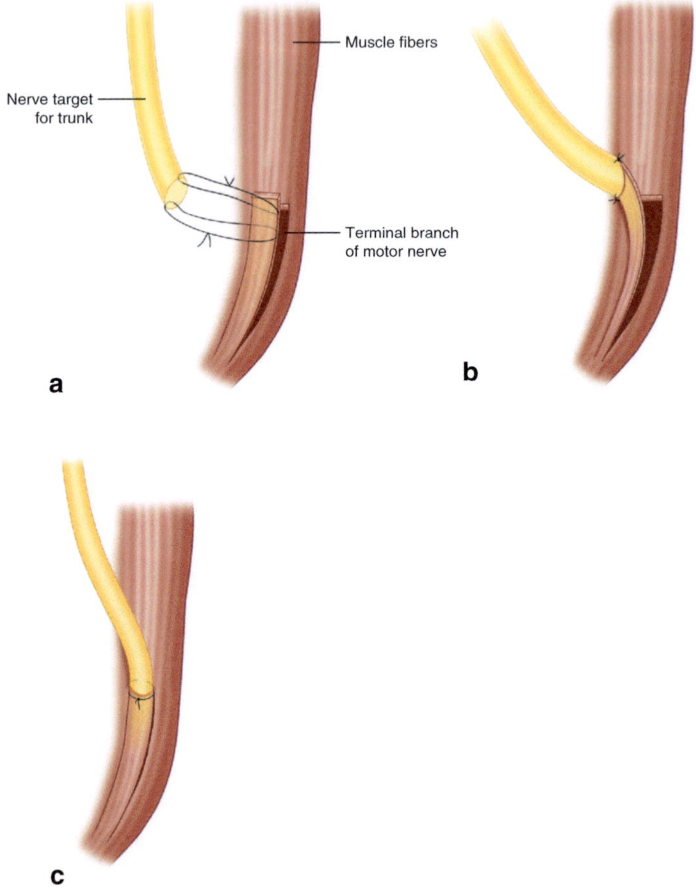

FIGURE 16.2 Schematic drawing of a nerve transfer before coaptation (**a**), after coaptation (**b**), and following imbrication of denervated muscle fibers (**c**). Note the severe size mismatch between the two nerves

Hip Disarticulation

Traumatic hip disarticulations and transpelvic amputations are relatively uncommon, but there are important considerations in their management. Even though they represent a small number of amputees, the vast majority of hip disarticulation or transpelvic amputation patients will require lifelong care and will have significant issues with pain and quality of life, so prevention of pain and complications is paramount. The basic tenet of hip disarticulations is adequate soft tissue coverage of bony prominences with healthy soft tissue.

Surgical preparation for hip disarticulation relies largely on the soft tissue envelope available for closure. Surgical positioning in the lateral position will allow for adequate access to both the anterior and posterior neurovascular structures. Careful dissection of the femoral triangle is facilitated by using an anterior racket incision. The quadratus femoris, iliopsoas, obturator, and gluteus medius are approximated over the acetabulum to obliterate dead space and provide cushion [8].

Large named nerves that will be encountered include the lateral femoral cutaneous nerve, the femoral nerve and its branches, the sciatic nerve, and the obturator nerve. Large caliber nerves, such as the sciatic and femoral nerves, should be dissected through perineural planes to create smaller nerve pedicles for transfer. All nerve transfers (i.e., TMR) performed for hip disarticulations can typically be done through existing incisions.

Above-Knee Amputation (Transfemoral Amputation)

Above-knee amputation (AKA) is the second most commonly performed amputation of the lower extremity. The obvious (and important) distinction from below-knee amputation (BKA) is the loss of the knee joint, as well as reduction in residual stump length. Because the knee joint is lost, keeping as much residual limb length as possible becomes even more important, as this is the lever arm for the prosthesis. Any amputation leaving less than

5 cm of length distal to the trochanter is functionally treated as a hip disarticulation, further increasing the energy strain for the patient.

When planning an AKA, soft tissue flaps are designed to take the incision just anterior to the maximal weight-bearing portion of the amputation, allowing the bone to be covered by the myodesis of the quadriceps, hamstring, and adductor muscle groups. The flaps should be designed several centimeters distal to the planned cut end of the bone. In the supine position, the saphenous nerve is identified medially and transferred to a nearby motor nerve target, typically within one of the adductor muscles. Likewise, the lateral femoral cutaneous nerve can be identified and coapted laterally to a target within the vastus lateralis. Myodesis is performed using a permanent suture with an inside-to-outside technique, which leaves the suture knots within the medullary canal. This technique will prevent abduction of the femur after amputation and allows for normal biomechanics with ambulation. Skin and fascia are closed in layers over a closed suction drain. Incisional negative pressure wound therapy (NPWT) is used for most patients undergoing AKA and TMR [4].

For the sciatic nerve and posterior femoral cutaneous nerves (PFCN), a separate longitudinal incision is used after the patient is placed in the prone position. The PFCN is identified suprafascially during the dissection toward the sciatic nerve. It should be noted that prior to closure of the fishmouth incision, it is important to liberate and tag the sciatic nerve so it can easily be dissected and delivered into the operative site for TMR. The sciatic nerve should be split into at least its peroneal and tibial subcomponents along perineural planes before it is transferred to identified motor nerve targets within the biceps femoris, semitendinosus, or semimembranosus muscles (Fig. 16.3). No drain is typically needed for this posterior incision, as minimal undermining is necessary and closure is performed in layers to obliterate dead space.

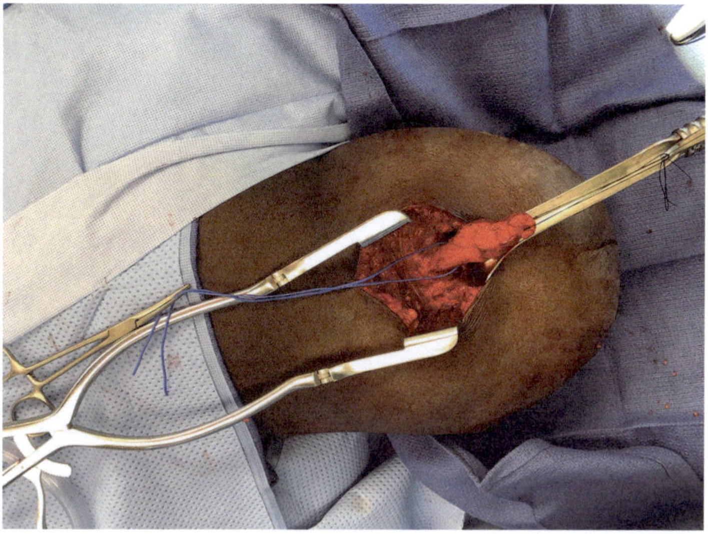

FIGURE 16.3 A large sciatic nerve neuroma is identified in a revision above-knee amputation. This nerve was split into two nerve pedicles and transferred separately

Below-Knee Amputation (Transtibial Amputation)

If a below-knee amputation (BKA) is required, several considerations should be taken into account. The skin incision most commonly used is based upon a posterior myocutaneous flap. The ideal flap gives adequate soft tissue coverage over the bone and also minimizes weight bearing directly on the incision line itself, when possible.

The suggested tibial bone length should be approximately 15 cm as measured from the tibial plateau, with an absolute minimum bone length being just beyond the tibial tubercle. Amputations proximal to the tibial tubercle lack flexion, and conversion to a higher-level amputation is likely. The fibula should be resected to a bone cut level at least 1–2 cm more proximal than the corresponding tibial transection level. Some authors advocate for an "Ertl Bridge," in which a cut portion of fibula is interposed between the tibia and fibula, with fixation with a syndesmotic screw. This procedure theoretically reduces soft tissue shearing from the underlying bony structure and forms a platform for stabilization and reduction in scissoring of the tibia and fibula bones [9].

During the dissection, it is important to identify the neurovascular bundles of the lower leg. In contrast to prior teaching, the major peripheral nerves should be identified and dissected distally to preserve as much length as possible. The tibial nerve, the common peroneal nerve (which, depending on the bone length, may be split into its deep and superficial branches), the saphenous nerve, and the sural nerve ideally should be identified for transfer in TMR surgery cases (Fig. 16.4). The tibial nerve is often large enough that it may

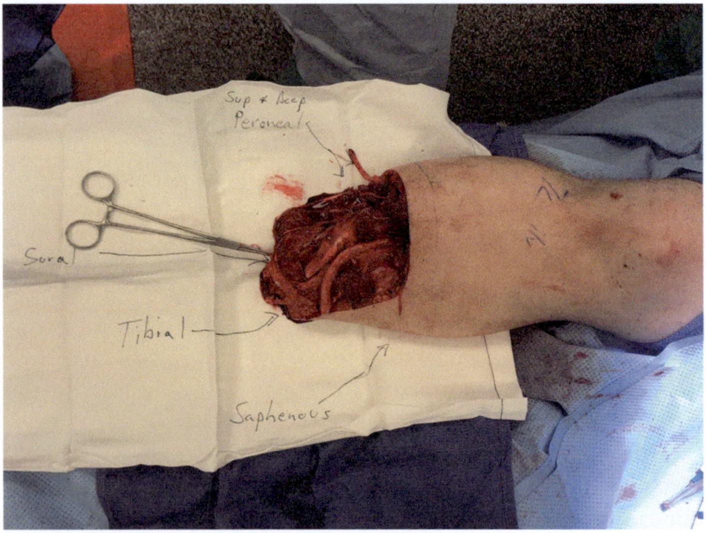

Figure 16.4 Nerve targets dissected and labeled during a below-knee amputation with immediate targeted muscle reinnervation (TMR). Note that the nerve pedicles have been dissected longer than the amputation to allow for greater freedom of mobility

be split along its perineural planes to create two smaller nerve pedicles for transfer. Tibial nerve transfer, as well as other nerve transfers, should be done at a level above the cut end of the bone to avoid pistoning of the bone onto the transferred nerves during ambulation. The nerve monitor will help identify terminal motor branches in the vicinity of the nerve pedicles as targets, being mindful to try to reinnervate each pedicle to different muscles. Of note, when performing TMR secondarily for BKA patients, it is often necessary to make separate posterior and more proximal incisions behind or above the knee to gain access to the nerves for transfer, as prior traction neurectomies result in the nerves being more proximally located within the residual limb.

Amputations of the Foot

Partial foot amputations can be quite problematic. They inherently create an imbalance in forces that can create pressure points that may be prone to ulceration. The choice of procedure for a partial foot amputation varies greatly based on the degree of viable tissue, premorbid vascular disease, biomechanics, and patient preferences. In some cases, a higher-level amputation (such as BKA) may be preferred because of the aforementioned factors.

Transmetatarsal, transtarsal, and tarsal amputations are all possibilities for partial foot amputations. Each typically uses a fishmouth incision, with deference given to saving as much glabrous skin as possible for weight-bearing status. Tension-free closure and minimal periosteal elevation are essential to prevent wound-healing complications and heterotopic ossification [10].

Nerve targets for TMR include branches of the deep and superficial peroneal nerves as they are identified during dissection, as well as the medial and lateral plantar nerves and the tibial nerve distal to the tarsal tunnel. The distal nature of the foot and the inherent arborization of the sensory nerves in the foot make TMR more difficult in distal amputations, but the motor nerves to the intrinsic foot muscles are excellent options for muscle targets for TMR within the foot.

Summary

Amputation of an extremity is a common procedure performed for a variety of indications. Modifications in technique are required for amputations at different levels (as well as upper versus lower extremities) to achieve optimal prosthetic function but several overlapping principles should be followed. Management of the underlying residual bone, soft tissue management, and consideration of peripheral nerve handling can be applied through all levels of amputations.

References

1. Lavelle DG. Amputations of the lower extremity. In: Azar FM, Canale ST, Beaty JH, editors. Campbell's operative orthopaedics. 13th ed. Philadelphia: Elsevier; 2017.
2. Göktepe AS, Cakir B, Yilmaz B, Yazicioglu K. Energy expenditure of walking with prostheses: comparison of three amputation levels. Prosthetics Orthot Int. 2010;34:31–6.
3. Meier RH, Melton D. Ideal functional outcomes for amputation levels. Phys Med Rehabil Clin N Am. 2014;25:199–212.
4. Gottschalk F. The importance of soft tissue stabilization in transfemoral amputation: English version. Orthopade. 2016;45:S1–4.
5. Kuiken TA, Dumanian GA, Lipschutz RD, Miller LA, Stubblefield KA. The use of targeted muscle reinnervation for improved myoelectric prosthesis control in a bilateral shoulder disarticulation amputee. Prosthetics Orthot Int. 2004;28:245–53.
6. Souza JM, Cheesborough JE, Ko JH, Cho MS, Kuiken TA, Dumanian GA. Targeted muscle reinnervation: a novel approach to postamputation neuroma pain. Clin Orthop Relat Res. 2014;472:2984–90.

7. Bowen JB, Wee CE, Kalik J, Valerio IL. Targeted muscle reinnervation to improve pain, prosthetic tolerance, and bioprosthetic outcomes in the amputee. Adv Wound Care (New Rochelle). 2017;6:261–7.
8. Wakelin SJ, Oliver CW, Kaufman MH. Hip disarticulation – the evolution of a surgical technique. Injury. 2004;35:299–308.
9. Chiodo CP, Stroud CC. Optimal surgical preparation of the residual limb for prosthetic fitting in below-knee amputations. Foot Ankle Clin. 2001;6:253–64.
10. Garwood CS, Steinberg JS. Soft tissue balancing after partial foot amputations. Clin Podiatr Med Surg. 2016;33:99–111.

Part II
Flap Atlas

Chapter 17
Soft Tissue Reconstruction of the Medial Thigh and Groin

Andrew L. Peredo, Victoria Wickenheisser, Caitlin Elizabeth Marks, and Scott T. Hollenbeck

Wounds in the groin region are very common. They are often secondary to vascular procedures and may involve exposed prosthetics [1]. Additionally, some of these patients have previously compromised peripheral vascular systems, so it is necessary to have a knowledge of a variety of flaps and their

A. L. Peredo
Department of Surgery, Division of Plastic and Reconstructive Surgery, University of Colorado, Anschutz Medical Campus, Aurora, CO, USA

V. Wickenheisser
Division of Plastic and Reconstructive Surgery, Duke University Hospital, Durham, NC, USA

C. E. Marks
Duke University School of Medicine, Duke University, Durham, NC, USA

S. T. Hollenbeck (✉)
Division of Plastic and Reconstructive Surgery, Duke University Medical Center, Durham, NC, USA
e-mail: scott.hollenbeck@duke.edu

S. T. Hollenbeck et al. (eds.), *Handbook of Lower Extremity Reconstruction*, https://doi.org/10.1007/978-3-030-41035-3_17

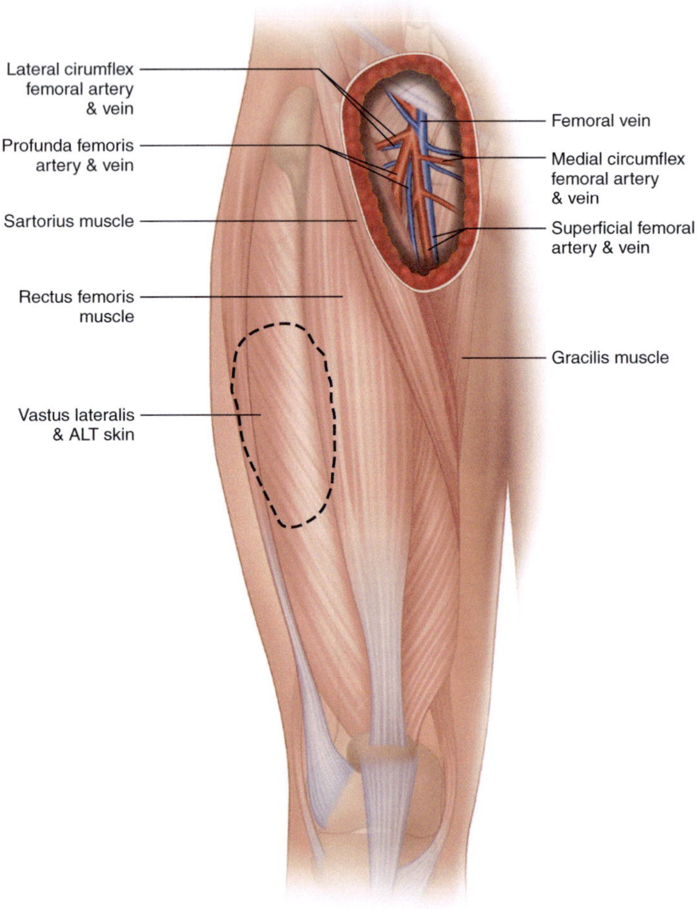

Figure 17.1 A complex groin wound with exposed femoral vessels. Potential flaps that are shown include the sartorius flap, gracilis flap, rectus femoris flap, and the anterolateral thigh (ALT)/vastus lateralis flap

associated vascular supply (Fig. 17.1). Likewise, wounds in the medial thigh, groin, and perineum are commonly related to oncologic resections. This chapter is specifically focused on groin wounds, but the same principles can apply to wounds of the medial thigh and some perineal wounds.

Overview of the Sartorius Flap

The sartorius flap is a type IV muscle flap. Its vascular origins are segmental branches of the superficial femoral artery. The muscle can be divided on a segmental branch to create a flap that can be positioned into the groin [2]. The muscle is relatively narrow and thin; it does not provide significant bulk or a skin component.

Markings for the Sartorius Flap

When used to cover groin defects, the sartorius flap is typically elevated and rotated from within the groin wound itself (Fig. 17.2). Typically, no skin paddle is used with this flap, so no specific skin markings are required, other than an extension of the groin wound.

Sartorius Flap Elevation

The sartorius flap is first identified within the wound bed. At the level of the groin, the muscle will typically be lateral to the femoral vessels. To see the muscle, the wound must be extended inferiorly and laterally. Once the muscle is visualized, the planned area for cutting can be anticipated (Fig. 17.3). Ultimately the muscle division will depend on the exact location of the segmental branches (Fig. 17.4).

Wound Closure

Once the sartorius muscle has been rotated into position, it may be sutured in place to adjacent connective tissue so that it lies directly over the exposed vessels. The skin defect may be partially closed, but often it is not amenable to primary closure. If the wound is now flush with the skin, a skin graft may be placed over the muscle (Fig. 17.5). If the defect is deep, packing over the muscle may be needed. A drain is usually placed in the region.

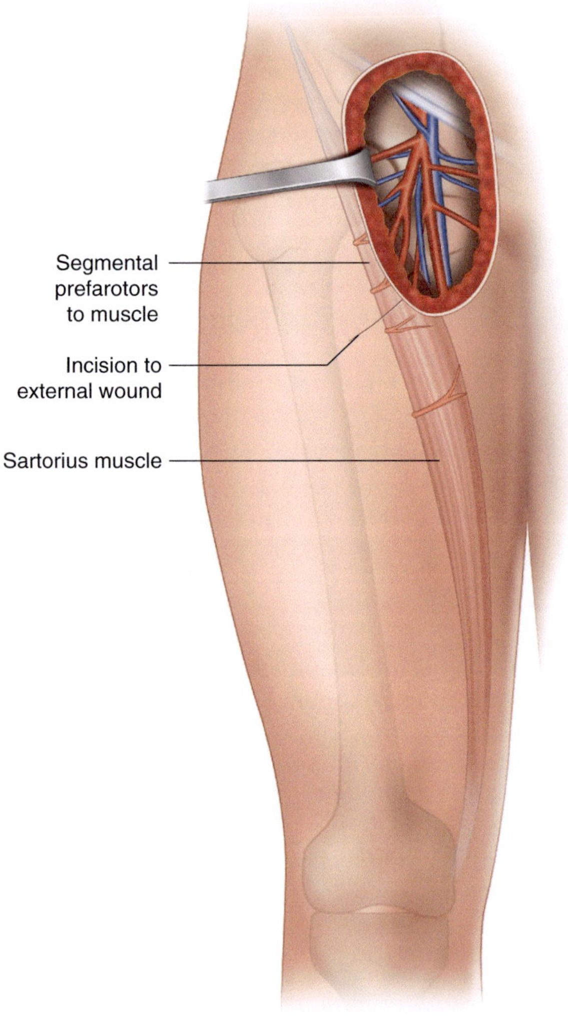

FIGURE 17.2 Sartorius flap for groin coverage. The groin wound extends down to the level of the femoral vessels. The sartorius muscle, which has segmental branches from the superficial femoral artery, can be identified at the lateral aspect of the groin wound as the most superficial muscle. The wound may need to be made larger by extending the skin incision inferior and laterally to eventually allow for good exposure of the sartorius muscle

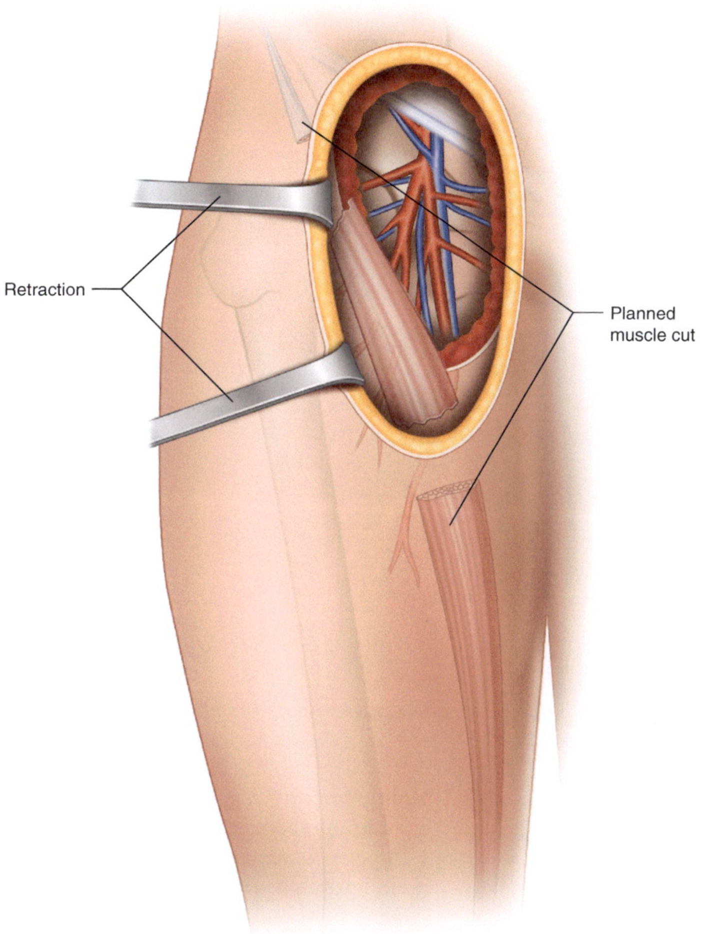

Figure 17.3 Dissection of the sartorius flap. With the wound extended, the sartorius muscle can be easily visualized with lateral traction. At this point, the segmental vascular branches must be found in order to plan how to divide the muscle such that it will have sufficient reach into the wound

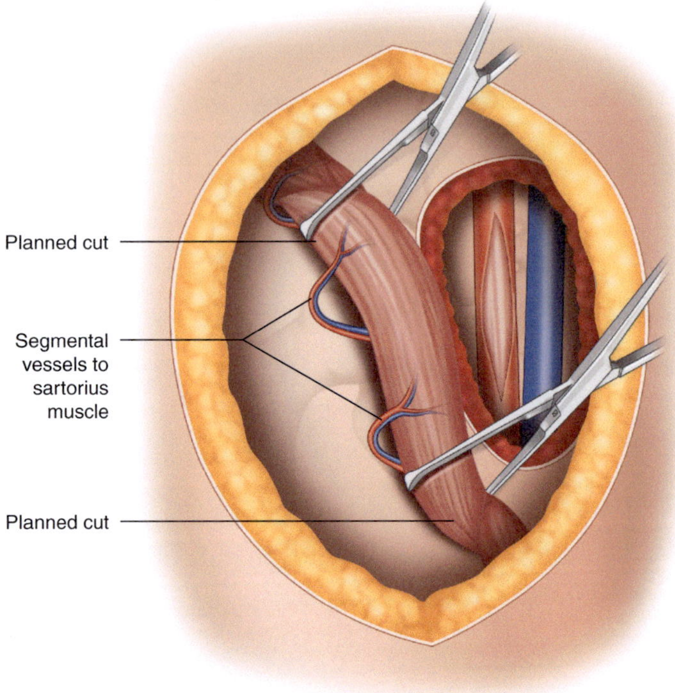

FIGURE 17.4 Dissection of the sartorius muscle flap. To visualize the segmental vascular branches into the sartorius muscle, the muscle may need to be reflected medially to flip it over. Based on the arc of rotation needed and the positioning of the segmental branches, two vessels may be kept intact in order to keep a relatively large piece of muscle for viable coverage. The muscle is then divided between two adjacent vascular branches and rotated into the defect (typically through eversion)

Overview of the Gracilis Flap

The gracilis is a type II muscle flap. Its vascular origin is the medial circumflex femoral artery, a branch of the profunda femoris vessels. The pedicle enters the muscle within the proximal one third of the muscle, along its medial aspect. A

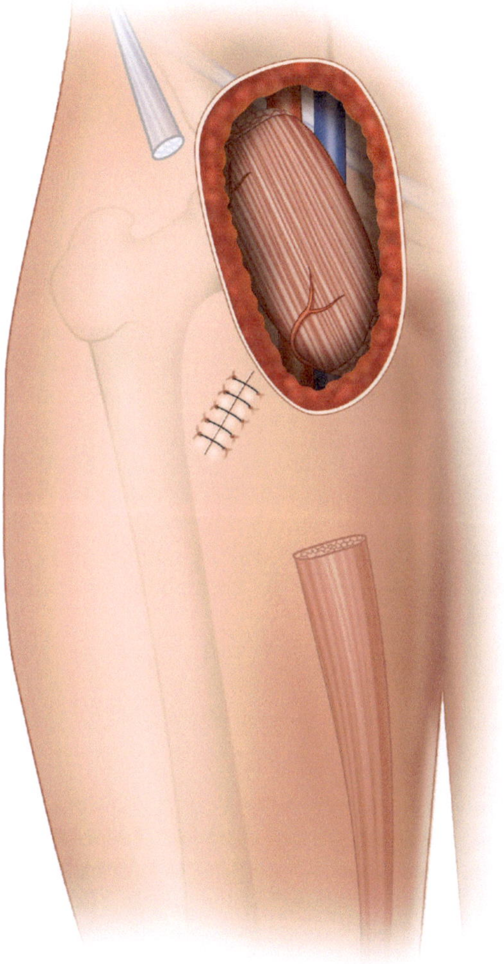

FIGURE 17.5 Closure of a groin defect with a sartorius flap. The muscle is placed over the femoral vessels, and a skin graft is performed or packing is placed

minor pedicle originating from the superficial femoral vessels enters the muscle more distally. For the purpose of groin wound closure, the gracilis muscle is usually divided distally and rotated into position to cover the femoral vessels or lymphatic leak.

Markings for the Gracilis Flap

The patient should be positioned supine with the hip abducted and knee flexed. The landmarks for the gracilis muscle are the adductor longus tendon as it leaves the ischiopubic ramus and the medial aspect of the knee. The gracilis muscle can be found slightly posterior and superficial to the adductor longus muscle.

The gracilis muscle origin is located just below the adductor longus origin on the pubic tuberosity. The distal gracilis tendon passes behind the medial femoral condyle and inserts in the upper medial tibia below the medial tibial condyle. A line drawn just posterior to the abductor longus to the medial tibial condyle indicates the location of the gracilis (Fig. 17.6).

Gracilis Flap Elevation

The medial circumflex femoral artery enters the gracilis muscle approximately 10 cm distal to the point of origin at the tubercle. The anterior branch of the obturator nerve supplies motor function to the gracilis muscle. The nerve courses obliquely from a cleft between the adductor longus and magnus muscles, entering the gracilis muscle just proximal to the medial circumflex femoral vessels.

When dissecting through the thigh fascia, take note of the marked line from the origin and insertion of the gracilis to avoid erroneous inclusion of the sartorius muscle or adductor longus (Figs. 17.7 and 17.8). Once the gracilis muscle fascia is identified, dissect the posterior edge of the gracilis muscle off the abductor magnus. Several minor vascular branches will require ligation on the anterior and posterior edge. Ensure

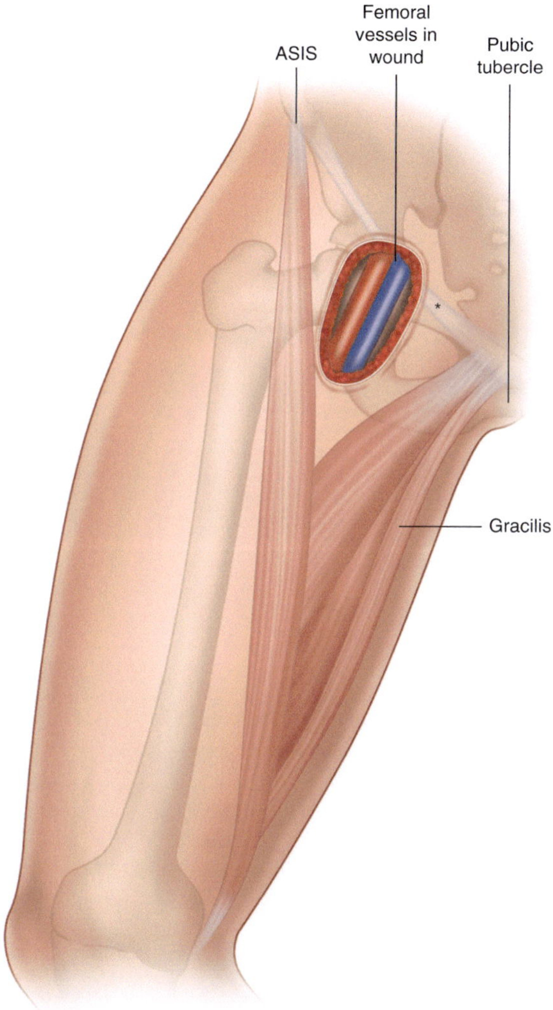

FIGURE 17.6 Markings for a gracilis flap for groin wound closure. The gracilis muscle can be found by first palpating for the adductor longus tendon along the medial aspect of the thigh (*asterisk*). A line can be drawn from that point to the medial aspect of the knee to guide the incision. The gracilis muscle will be just posterior to the adductor longus and just anterior to the adductor magnus. ASIS—anterior superior iliac spine

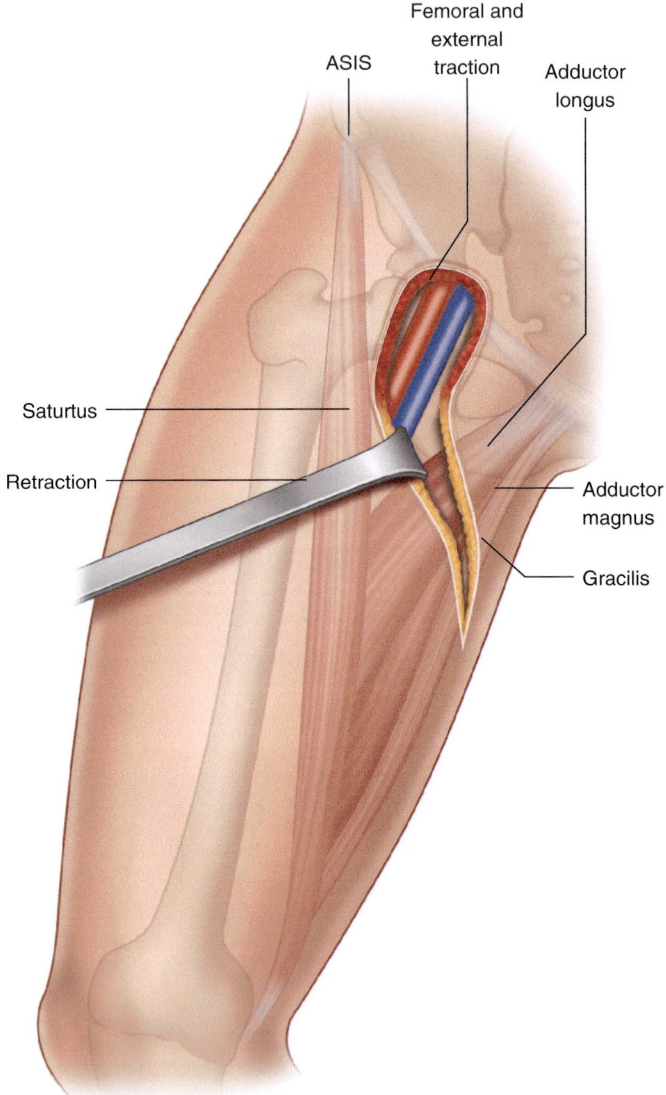

FIGURE 17.7 Elevation of gracilis flap. The wound has been extended to allow for visualization of the gracilis muscle. The planned distal cut in the muscle is seen. Retraction is required to see the distal aspect of the muscle

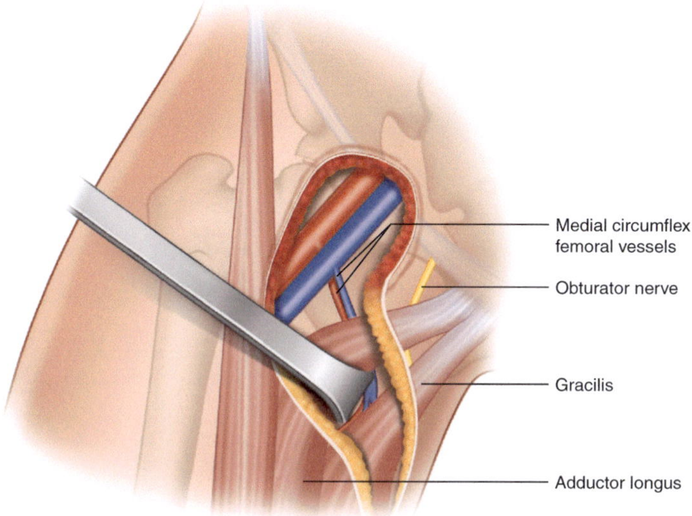

FIGURE 17.8 Isolation of the gracilis muscle on its vascular pedicle. The gracilis muscle can be gently retracted away from the adductor muscles to allow for visualization of the medial circumflex femoral vessels. The obturator nerve (*yellow*) is also seen entering the muscle along its proximal and medial aspect

that the dominant pedicle is verified prior to ligating any branches. The muscle can then be distally divided and rotated as needed.

Wound Closure

Once the gracilis muscle has been rotated into position, it may be sutured in place to adjacent connective tissue so that it lies directly over the exposed vessels (Fig. 17.9). The skin defect may be partially closed, but often it is not amenable to primary closure. If the wound is now flush with the skin, a skin graft can be placed over the muscle. If the defect is deep, then packing over the muscle may be needed. A drain is usually placed in the region.

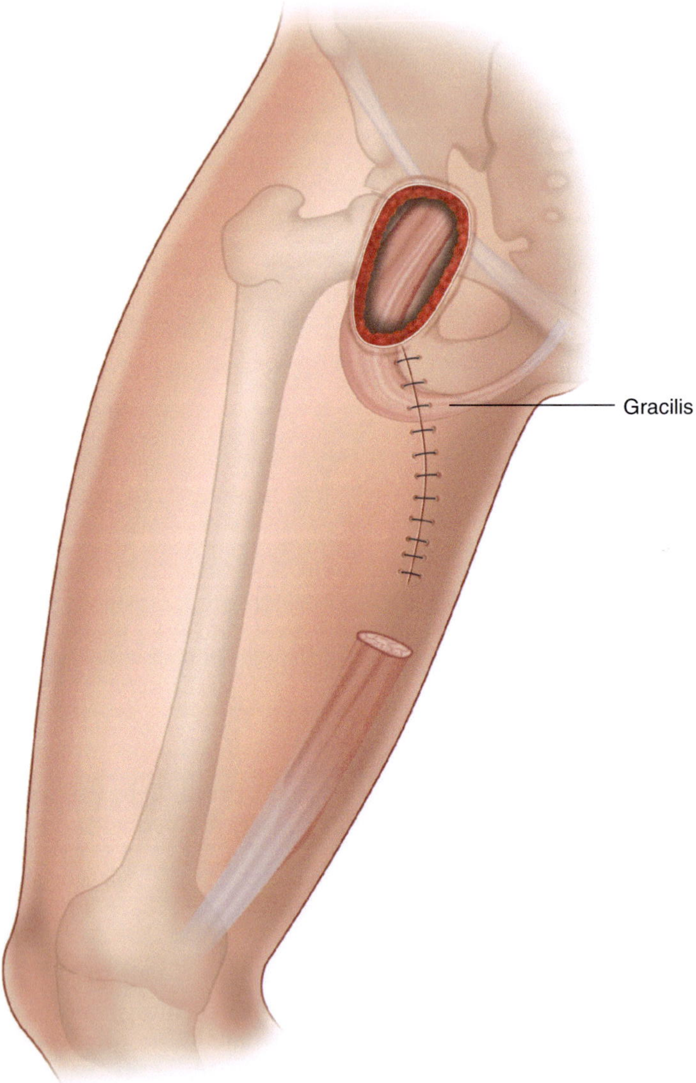

FIGURE 17.9 Gracilis flap closure of groin wound. The gracilis muscle is divided distally and rotated to cover the femoral vessels

Overview of the Rectus Femoris Flap

The rectus femoris is a type II muscle flap and can be very useful for groin defects [3]. Its vascular origin is the lateral circumflex femoral artery, a branch of the profunda femoris vessels. The pedicle enters the muscle within the proximal one third of the muscle, along its lateral aspect. A minor pedicle originating from the superficial femoral vessels enters the muscle more distally. For the purpose of groin wound closure, the rectus femoris muscle is usually divided distally and rotated into position to cover the femoral vessels or lymphatic leak. Skin from the anterior thigh can be included reliably with the flap.

Markings for the Rectus Femoris Flap

The patient should be positioned supine. The landmarks for the rectus femoris muscle are a line drawn from the anterior superior iliac spine (ASIS) to the center of the patella (Fig. 17.10). A skin island can be designed within the proximal mid thigh, along this line. The rectus femoris muscle lies directly below the skin and superficial fascia and is easily identified.

Rectus Femoris Flap Elevation

The muscle is directly below the skin and fascia of the mid thigh. The lateral circumflex femoral artery gives a branch that enters the rectus femoris muscle along its undersurface at the proximal and lateral aspect of the muscle. Whichever skin incision is used must allow for adequate visualization of the pedicle to prevent injury and twisting during flap elevation. The distal aspect of the rectus femoris is divided either through a counter-incision (Fig. 17.11) or by extending the skin incision down the leg.

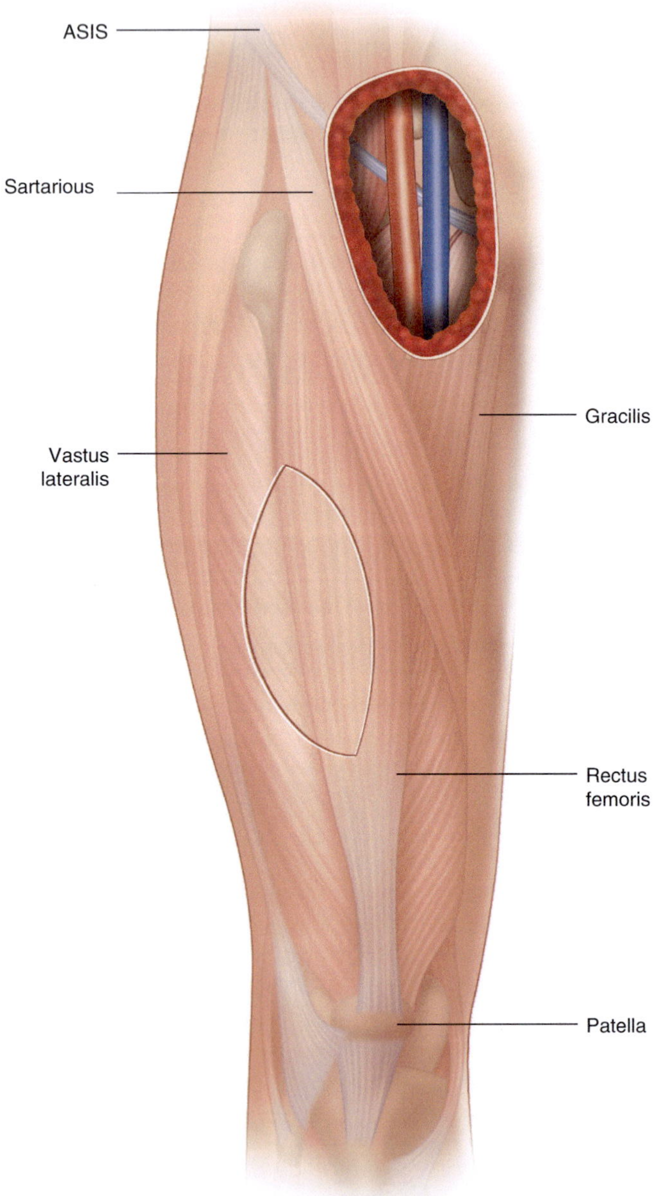
ASIS
Sartarious
Vastus lateralis
Gracilis
Rectus femoris
Patella

FIGURE 17.10 Markings for a rectus femoris flap for groin wound closure. The rectus femoris muscle can be found in the mid-thigh, directly below a line drawn between the anterior superior iliac spine (ASIS) and the central patella. There are several options for the incision. If both skin and muscle will be used, a skin island can be designed over the muscle. If only muscle is to be used, an extension of the groin wound can be used to see the proximal muscle; it can be extended down the leg for further exposure (*dashed line*). Another option is to make a counter-incision to expose the distal muscle for division

Wound Closure

Once the rectus femoris muscle has been rotated into position, it may be sutured in place to adjacent connective tissue so that it lies directly over the exposed vessels. The skin defect can be primarily closed or skin grafted (Fig. 17.12). If the wound is now flush with the skin, a skin graft may be placed over the muscle. If the defect is deep, then packing over the muscle may be needed. If skin has been included in the flap, then the groin wound may be definitively closed. A drain is usually placed in the region.

Overview of the ALT Flap

The anterolateral thigh (ALT) flap is a versatile fasciocutaneous flap that can be used for medial or lateral thigh defects, as further discussed in Chap. 18 [4]. The flap can also include a portion of the vastus lateralis muscle to add bulk.

Markings for the ALT Flap

When used to cover groin defects, the ALT flap typically is elevated and rotated towards the defect. To do so, the flap and its pedicle must be passed underneath the rectus femoris muscle. A skin island of sufficient size to close the groin

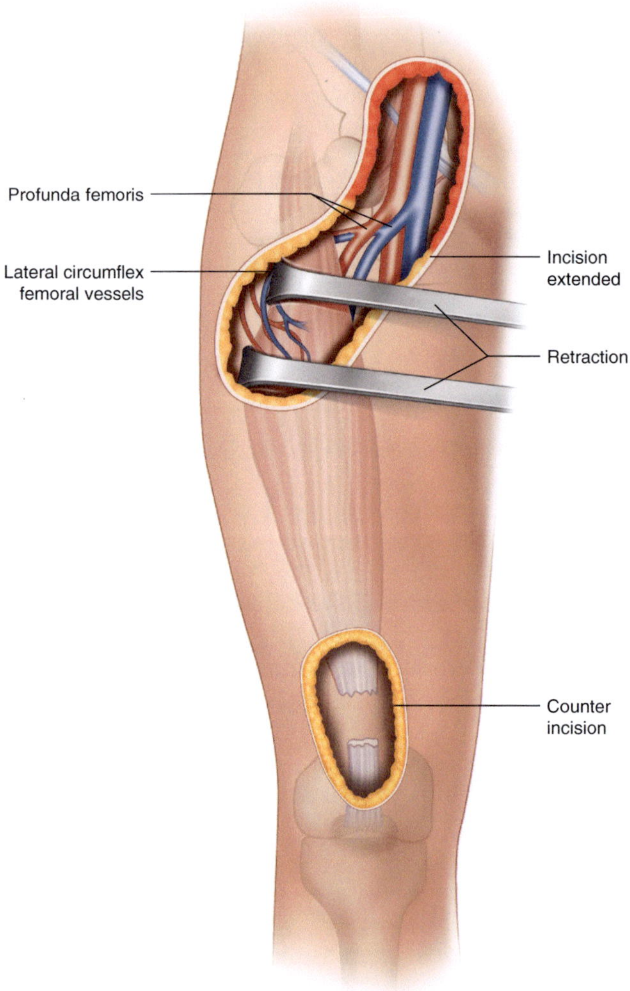

Figure 17.11 Elevation of rectus femoris muscle flap. The wound has been extended to allow for visualization of the rectus femoris muscle. The muscle has been partially retracted medially for visualization of the pedicle from the lateral circumflex femoral vessels. A counter-incision is shown, which allows for division of the distal muscle

wound can be designed (Fig. 17.13). With the patient in the supine position, a line is drawn from the anterior superior iliac spine (ASIS) to the superolateral aspect of the patella. At the mid-point of this line, perforators to the ALT skin flap typically can be defined with a handheld Doppler or through direct visualization during flap elevation.

ALT Flap Elevation

The ALT flap is raised along the medial aspect to first identify perforators. Several perforators may be included in the flap as they originate off the descending branch of the lateral circumflex femoral artery (LCFA). Some of these perforators may run in the septum between the vastus lateralis and the rectus femoris; others may traverse the vastus lateralis muscle for some distance (Fig. 17.14). The remainder of the skin can be elevated once the perforators are found. The distal aspect of the descending branch of the LCFA is then ligated, which allows the proximal portion of the vessels and the flap to be passed under the rectus femoris muscle to reach the groin.

Wound Closure

Once the ALT flap has been rotated into position, it may be sutured in place to adjacent connective tissue so that it lies directly over the exposed vessels. The groin wound may be closed with the skin of the ALT flap. The donor site is closed either primarily or with a split-thickness skin graft (Fig. 17.15). A drain is usually placed in the region.

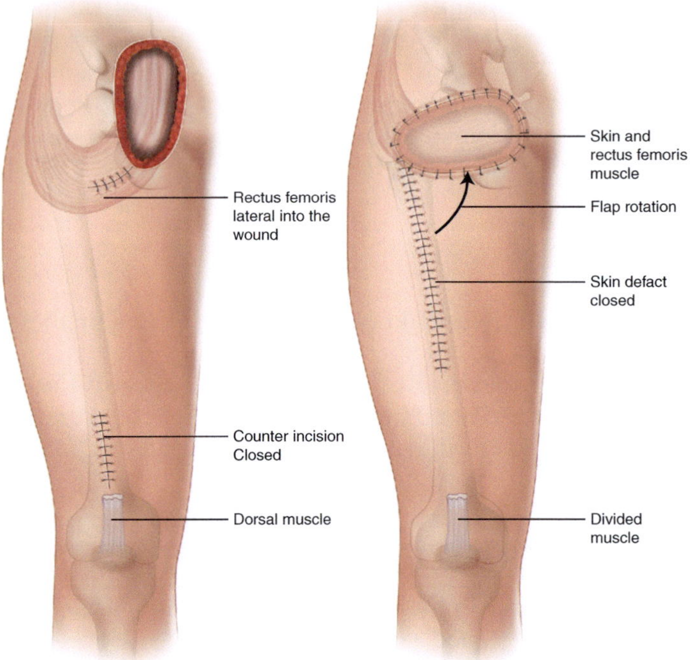

FIGURE 17.12 Rectus femoris flap closure of groin wound. *Left,* The rectus femoris muscle is divided distally and rotated to cover the femoral vessels. *Right,* A rectus femoris flap including a skin island has been rotated to close the groin wound. The donor site has been closed primarily

FIGURE 17.13 Markings for an ALT flap for groin wound closure. The ALT flap can be designed based on perforators from the descending branch of the lateral circumflex femoral vessels. The perforators are centered on a line drawn from the ASIS to the lateral aspect of the patella. A skin island can be designed around the perforators. A proximal extension of the incision may be necessary to visualize the flap pedicle

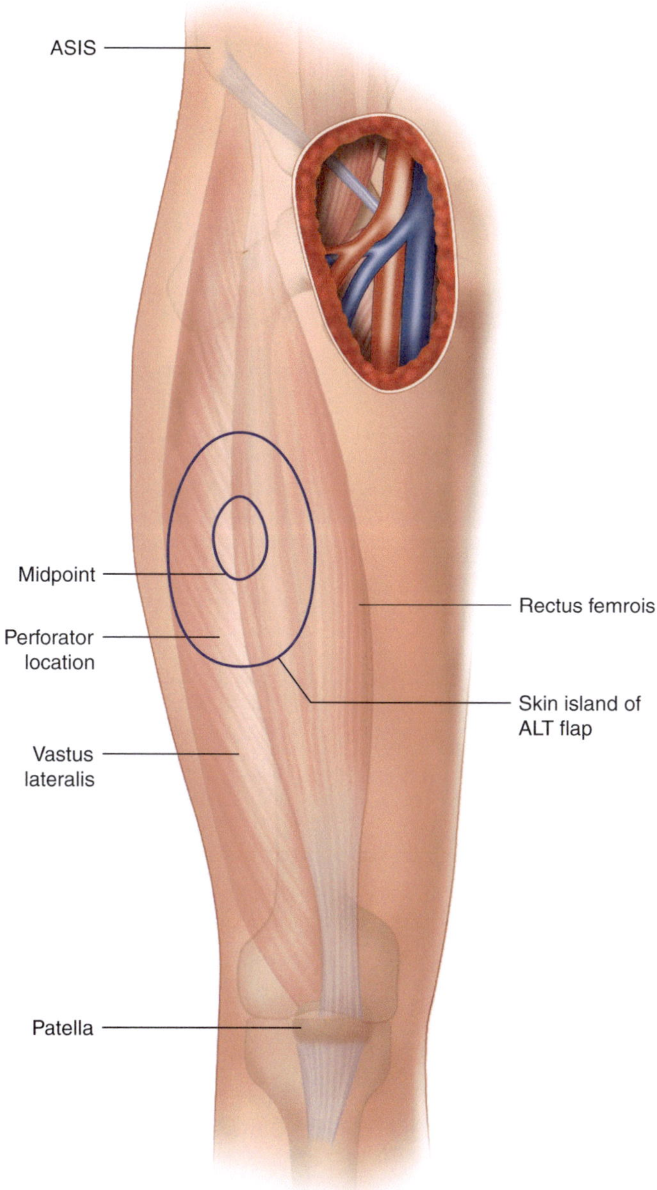
ASIS
Midpoint
Perforator location
Vastus lateralis
Patella
Rectus femrois
Skin island of ALT flap

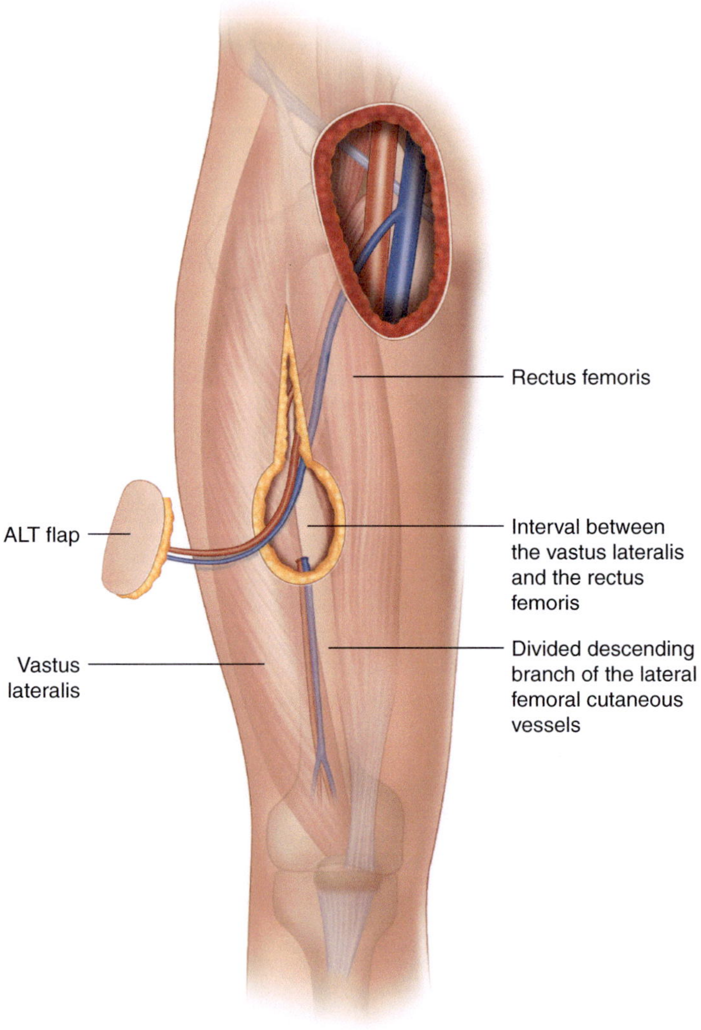

Figure 17.14 Elevation of ALT flap. The ALT flap has been elevated off the underlying muscles. The flap pedicle is dissected in the interval between the rectus femoris muscle and vastus lateralis muscle

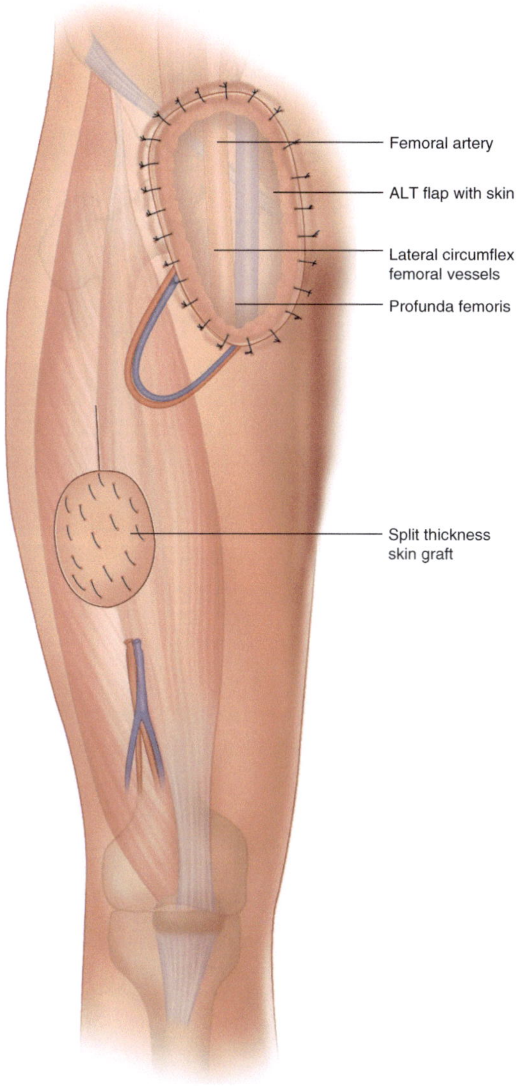

FIGURE 17.15 ALT flap closure of groin wound. The ALT flap and its pedicle are passed under the rectus femoris to allow for direct placement into the groin wound and closure. The donor site is closed with a split-thickness skin graft

References

1. Morasch MD, Sam AD, Kibbe MR, Hijjawi G, Dumanian GA. Early results with use of gracilis muscle flap coverage of infected groin wounds after vascular surgery. J Vasc Surg. 2004;39:1277–83.
2. Wu LC, Djohan RS, Liu TS, Chao AH, Lohman RF, Song DH. Proximal vascular pedicle preservation for Sartorius muscle flap transposition. Plast Reconstr Surg. 2006;117(1):253–8.
3. Alkon JD, Smith A, Losee JE, Illig KA, Green RM, Serletti JM. Management of complex groin wounds: preferred use of the rectus femoris muscle flap. Plast Reconstr Surg. 2005;115(3):776–83.
4. LoGiudice JA, Haberman K, Sanger JR. The anterolateral thigh flap for groin and lower abdominal defects: a better alternative to the rectus abdominis flap. Plast Reconstr Surg. 2014;133(1):162–8.

Chapter 18
Soft Tissue Reconstruction of the Lateral Thigh and Hip

Mahsa Taskindoust and Scott T. Hollenbeck

Wounds that overlie the greater trochanter are common and at times require flap coverage. Two local flaps are well suited for these defects. The tensor fascia lata (TFL) flap and the anterolateral thigh (ALT) flap both have vascular origins from the lateral circumflex femoral artery and can be positioned proximally for hip coverage (Fig. 18.1).

M. Taskindoust
Levine Science Research Center, Duke University, Durham, NC, USA

S. T. Hollenbeck (✉)
Division of Plastic and Reconstructive Surgery, Duke University Medical Center, Durham, NC, USA
e-mail: scott.hollenbeck@duke.edu

S. T. Hollenbeck et al. (eds.), *Handbook of Lower Extremity Reconstruction*, https://doi.org/10.1007/978-3-030-41035-3_18

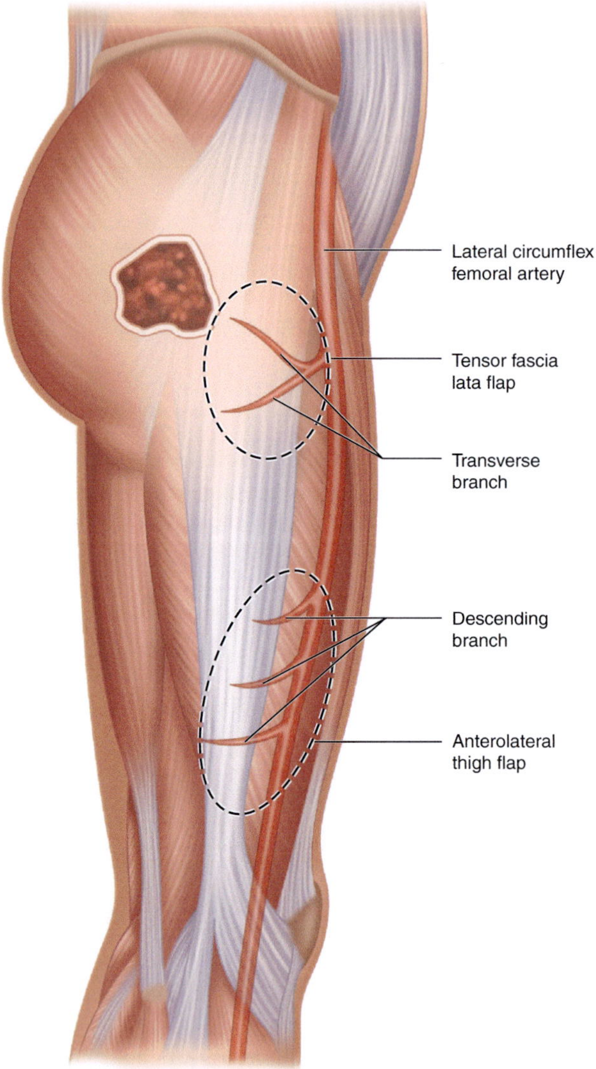

FIGURE 18.1 Lateral thigh/hip wound. This lateral view of the thigh and buttock shows a wound over the greater trochanter of the femur, with exposure of the bone. The two flaps most suited for covering it, the tensor fascia lata flap and the anterolateral thigh flap, both have vascular origins from the lateral circumflex femoral artery

Overview of the Tensor Fascia Lata (TFL) Flap

When used for coverage of the thigh and hip, the TFL flap is typically created as a myocutaneous flap. It can be also used for coverage of groin and midline defects when other options are not available.

Markings for the TFL Flap

When used to cover hip defects, the TFL flap typically is elevated and rotated or advanced towards the defect. In many instances, this can be done in a V to Y configuration.

TFL Flap Elevation

The TFL is raised from distal to proximal. The fascia lata can be included with the flap. The vascular pedicle is the transverse branch of the lateral circumflex femoral artery. The pedicle originates from the profunda femoris artery and enters the muscle along the proximal and medial aspect.

Wound Closure

The lateral thigh wound is closed with the proximal portion of the flap as it is advanced up the leg. The donor site can be closed in a primary manner (such as the V to Y) or with a split-thickness skin graft.

Overview of the Anterolateral Thigh (ALT) Flap

The ALT flap is a versatile fasciocutaneous flap that can be used for medial or lateral thigh defects. The flap can also include a portion of the vastus lateralis muscle to add bulk.

Markings for the ALT Flap

When used to cover hip defects, the ALT flap typically is elevated and rotated or advanced towards the defect, in a manner similar to the TFL. A large skin paddle can be created with the anticipation of sliding it up the leg towards the defect. If the flap is created as a V pattern, primary closure of the donor defect may be possible. With the patient in the supine position, a line is drawn from the anterior superior iliac spine (ASIS) to the superolateral aspect of the patella (Fig. 18.2). At the mid-point of this line, there are typically perforators to the ALT skin flap. These can be defined with a handheld Doppler. The distal part of the flap is designed as a V shape. The proximal portion of the flap extends to the hip wound.

ALT Flap Elevation

The ALT flap is raised along the medial aspect to first identify perforators. Several perforators may be included in the flap as they originate off the descending branch of the lateral circumflex femoral artery (LCFA) (Fig. 18.3). Some of these perforators may run in the septum between the vastus lateralis and the rectus femoris; others may traverse the vastus lateralis muscle for some distance. The remainder of the skin can be elevated once the perforators are found. The distal aspect of the LCFA is then ligated, allowing for the proximal portion of the vessels to be shifted up the leg towards the lateral thigh wound.

Wound Closure

The lateral thigh wound is closed with the proximal portion of the flap as it is advanced up the leg. The donor site can be closed in a primary manner, such as the V to Y (Fig. 18.4), or with a split-thickness skin graft.

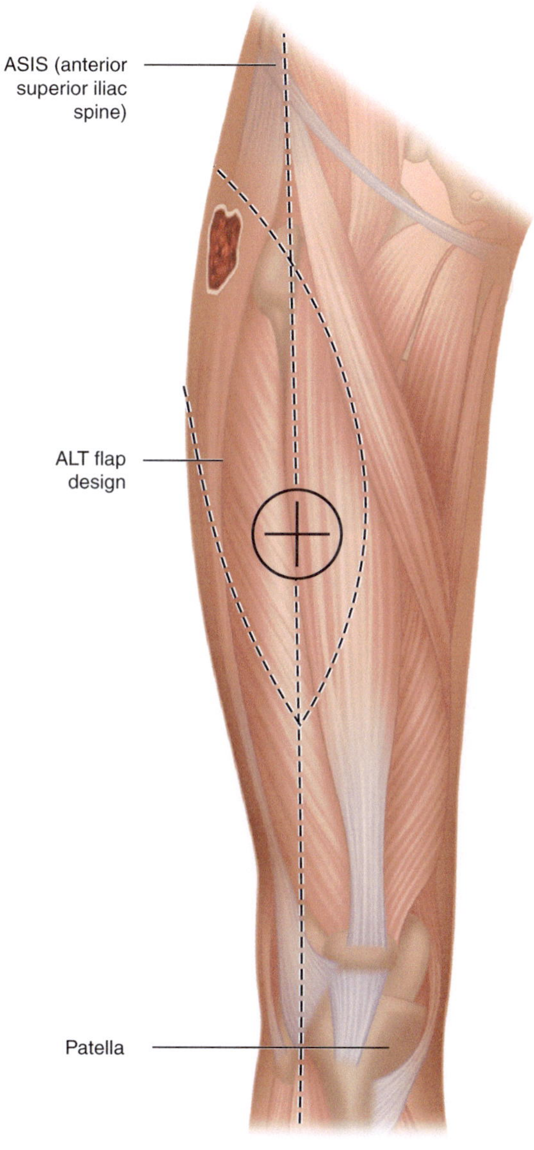

FIGURE 18.2 Markings for an anterolateral thigh (ALT) flap V to Y for closure of a hip wound

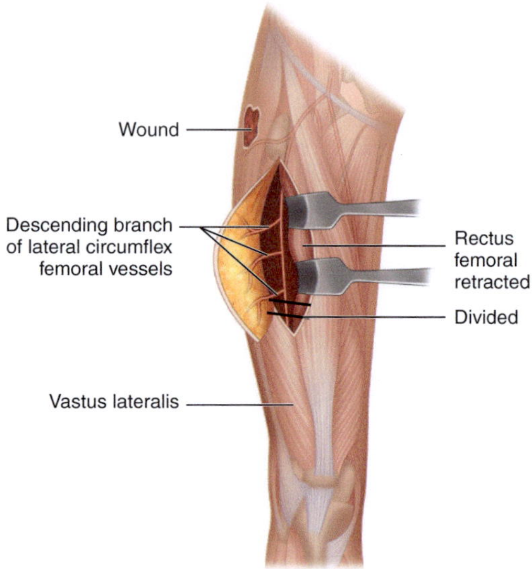

Figure 18.3 ALT flap elevation

Figure 18.4 ALT flap V to Y closure

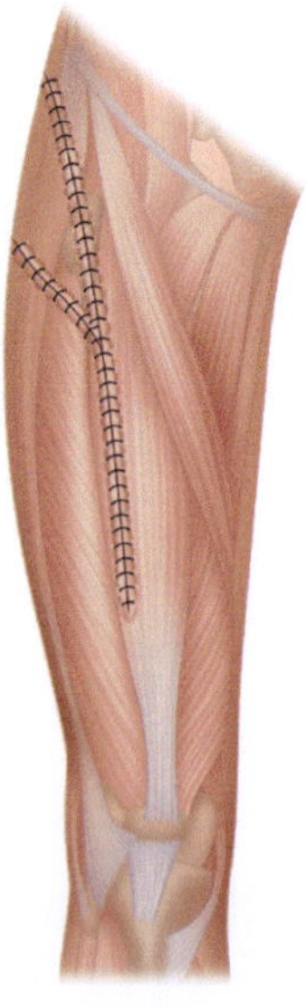

Suggested Reading

Zenn MR, Jones G. Thigh. In: Zenn MR, Jones G, editors. Reconstructive surgery: anatomy, technique, and clinical application. St. Louis: Quality Medical Publishing; 2012.

Chapter 19
Soft Tissue Reconstruction of the Distal Thigh and Proximal Knee

Victoria Wickenheisser and Scott T. Hollenbeck

Wounds in the upper knee region can occur after trauma, but they are typically associated with orthopedic procedures. They are often secondary to vascular procedures and may involve exposed prosthetics. The lower knee area is amenable to coverage with a gastrocnemius flap, but the upper knee is often out of the reach of this flap. In these circumstances, the reconstructive surgeon should be familiar with several other options (Fig. 19.1).

V. Wickenheisser
Division of Plastic and Reconstructive Surgery, Duke University Hospital, Durham, NC, USA

S. T. Hollenbeck (✉)
Division of Plastic and Reconstructive Surgery, Duke University Medical Center, Durham, NC, USA
e-mail: scott.hollenbeck@duke.edu

S. T. Hollenbeck et al. (eds.), *Handbook of Lower Extremity Reconstruction*, https://doi.org/10.1007/978-3-030-41035-3_19

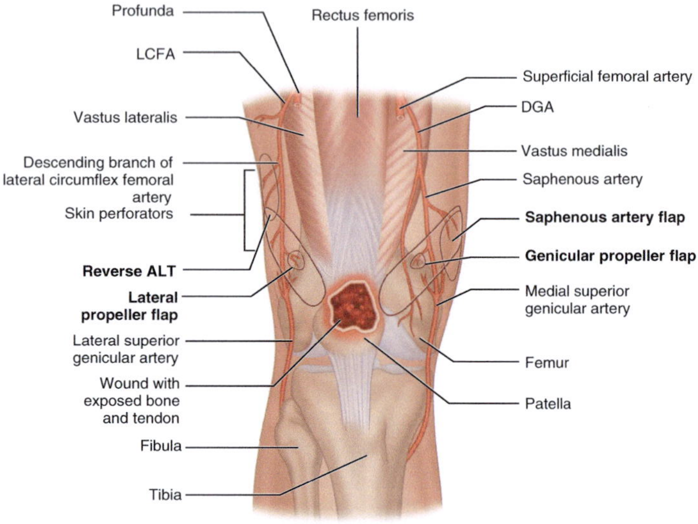

Figure 19.1 This wound in the upper knee area is associated with a prior linear incision for a total knee arthroplasty. A gastrocnemius flap will not reach this area. Options for this wound include the saphenous flap, the medial or lateral thigh propeller flap, and the reverse anterolateral thigh (ALT) flap

Overview of the Saphenous Flap

The saphenous flap is a fasciocutaneous flap with vascular origins at the saphenous artery originating from the descending genicular artery [1]. The saphenous artery will have a skin perforator that can be localized in the upper medial aspect of the knee.

Markings for the Saphenous Flap

When used to cover upper knee defects, the saphenous flap can be designed as a pedicle flap along the medial and upper aspect of the knee (Fig. 19.2).

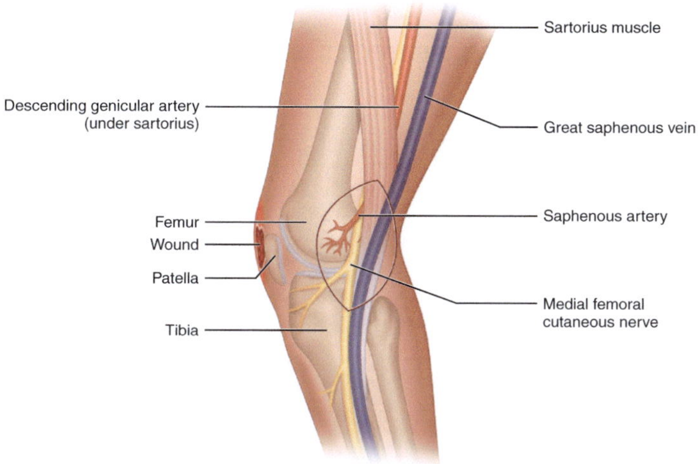

Figure 19.2 The saphenous flap for upper knee coverage is designed based on a skin perforator from the saphenous artery, which originates from the descending genicular artery. The primary pedicle will emerge from under the sartorius muscle, so a proximal extension of the incision over the sartorius will allow for visualization. The great saphenous vein and the medial circumflex femoral cutaneous nerve are near the pedicle and typically will be spared

Saphenous Flap Elevation

The saphenous flap is created by first finding the primary pedicle. The saphenous artery originates from the descending genicular artery, which runs under the sartorius muscle. The sartorius muscle can be reflected to visualize the pedicle and dissect it away from surrounding structures (Fig. 19.3). If the skin perforator is medial to the sartorius muscle, then the muscle will need to be split in order to transfer the flap to the knee. One alternative approach is to keep the proximal portion of the skin flap attached. In this instance, the flap will be transposed into the defect along the anterior leg.

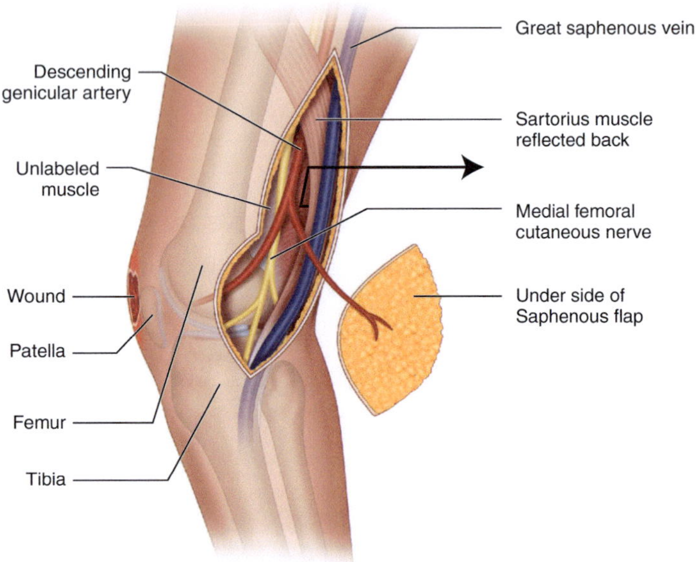

Figure 19.3 Dissection of the saphenous flap. The flap skin island has been raised, and the pedicle can be seen entering the flap. In order to see the primary descending genicular artery pedicle, the sartorius muscle must be reflected, along with the great saphenous vein. The medial femoral cutaneous nerve typically is spared during the dissection

Wound Closure

Once the saphenous flap has been elevated, it may be tunneled are transposed into position. A skin graft may be needed to close the donor defect.

Overview of the Medial and Lateral Thigh Propeller Flap

The propeller flap concept can be useful for defects in the lower thigh and upper knee [2]. Propeller flaps are fasciocutaneous flaps that are based on any available perforator. The perforator and pedicle must be of sufficient length after dissection to allow for a 180-degree turn without causing a twist or kink. The perforator should also be as close to the defect as possible to allow for favorable flap dimensions.

Markings for the Medial Thigh Propeller Flap

Once a perforator has been found with a Doppler probe or ultrasound device, the flap can be designed (Fig. 19.4). First the width of the wound is measured (length A). Then the distance from the perforator to the defect is measured (length B). The amount of proximal tissue needed will be that which reaches the defect after the 180 degree turn (length A + B). Ideally, the direction of the long arm of the limb would be consistent with known angiosome territories. It is often possible to carry the primary angiosome and a secondary angiosome with a propeller flap.

Medial Thigh Propeller Flap Elevation

Once a perforator has been identified and the flap dimensions have been marked, the skin incision can be made. The dissection will proceed down to the level of the muscle fascia. The perforator is then seen exiting the thigh muscles and entering the skin flap. The perforator should then be dissected as deep as possible, to gain sufficient length for the pedicle to be twisted 180 degrees without forming a kink (Fig. 19.5). Once the pedicle is sufficiently mobilized, the remainder of the flap is elevated. Finally, the flap is turned 180 degrees and the long arm will now be positioned over the defect.

Wound Closure

Once the propeller flap has been turned 180°, the defect can be closed with the long arm of the flap (Fig. 19.6). The short arm of the flap will partially cover the donor defect. The remaining defect may be closed primarily or with a skin graft. A drain is usually placed in the region.

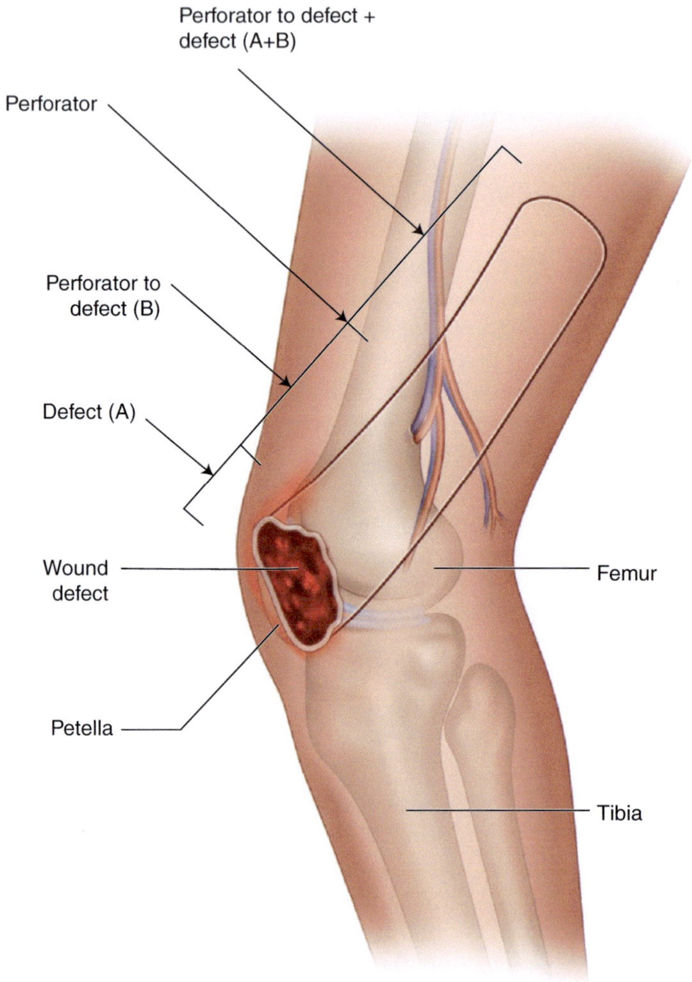

FIGURE 19.4 Markings for a medial thigh propeller flap to cover an upper knee defect. The flap is based on a perforator that is located close to the defect. The defect size is measured (length A). The distance from the perforator to the defect is measured (length B). The long arm of the flap is the same height as the defect, with a length sufficient to cover the defect (length A + B)

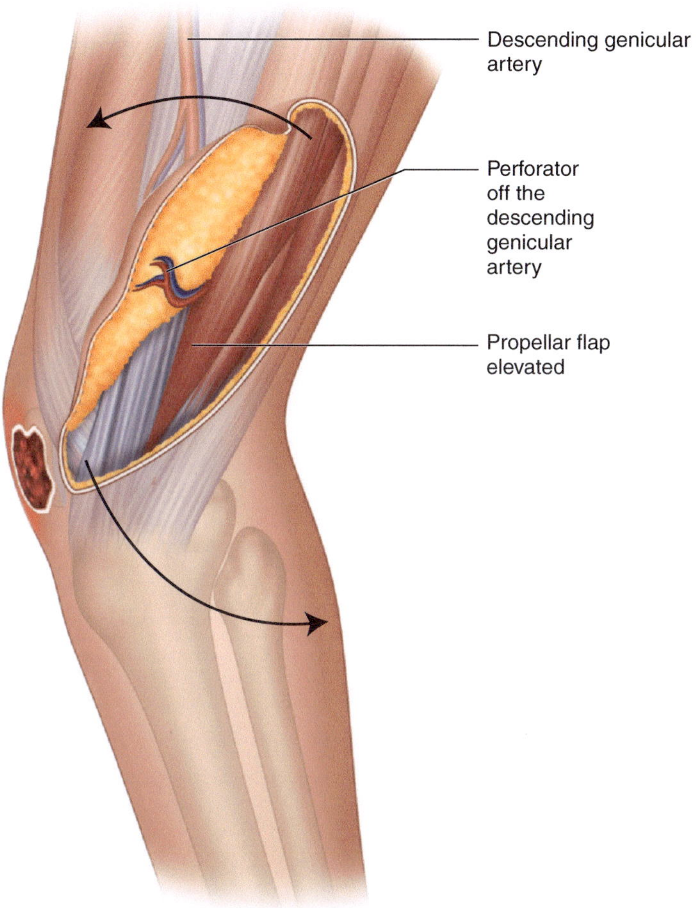

Figure 19.5 Elevation of the medial thigh propeller flap for a knee wound. The perforator of the flap is dissected back into the muscle to create sufficient length to avoid kinking

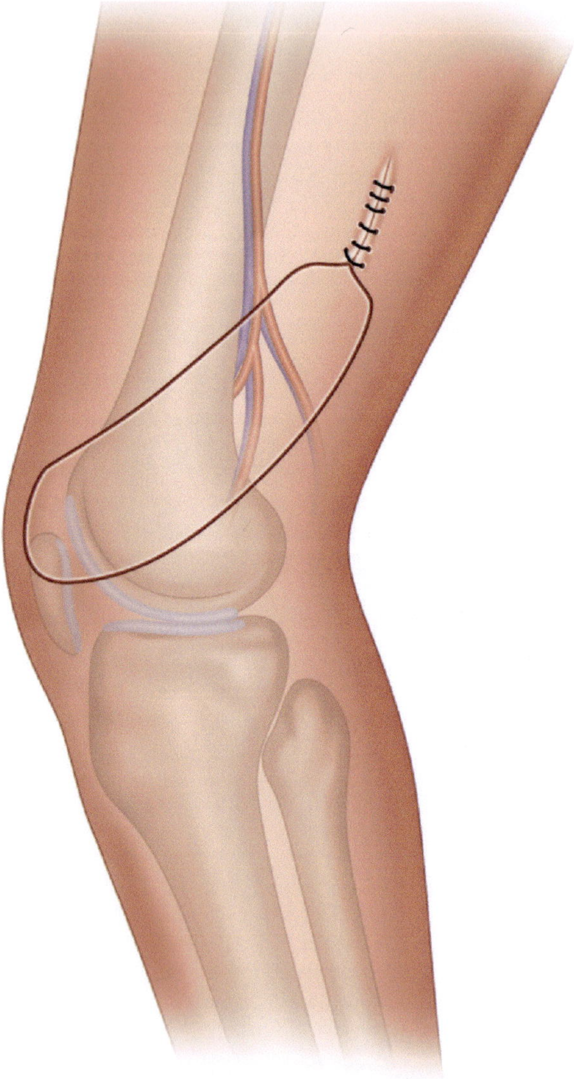

FIGURE 19.6 Medial thigh propeller flap closure. The flap has been turned 180 degrees, and the long arm has been used to close the defect. The short arm has been used to partially close the donor defect, with the remainder closed primarily. Note that the pedicle now has a 180-degree twist, but there is sufficient length to avoid kinking

Overview of the Reverse Anterolateral Thigh (ALT) Flap

The reverse ALT flap is useful for coverage of the lower thigh or upper knee, as well as the popliteal fossa [3]. The vascular origins are the perforators from the descending branch of the lateral circumflex femoral vessels; these perforators will receive *retrograde* flow from the lateral superior genicular vessels. The proximal lateral circumflex femoral vessels will be ligated to allow for distal transposition of the flap.

Markings for the Reverse ALT Flap

The markings for the reverse ALT are similar to those for a standard ALT flap. With the patient in the supine position, a line is drawn from the anterior superior iliac spine (ASIS) to the superolateral aspect of the patella. At the mid-point of this line, there are typically perforators to the ALT skin flap. These can be defined with a handheld Doppler or through direct visualization during flap elevation. If multiple perforators are available, a distal perforator is preferable, as it is closer to the inflow of the lateral superior genicular vessels (Fig. 19.7). A skin island of sufficient size to close the wound can be designed around the perforator.

Reverse ALT Flap Elevation

The reverse ALT flap is raised along the medial aspect to first identify perforators in a similar fashion to the standard ALT flap. Several perforators may be included in the flap as they originate off the descending branch of the lateral circumflex femoral artery (LCFA), but a distal perforator is most desirable. Some of these perforators may run in the septum between the vastus lateralis and the rectus femoris; others may traverse the vastus lateralis muscle for some distance.

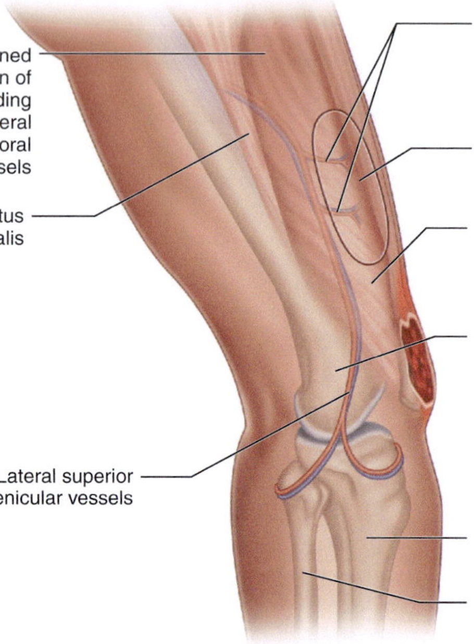

FIGURE 19.7 Markings for a reverse ALT flap for coverage of a wound on the distal thigh. The flap will be based on perforators from the lateral circumflex femoral vessels, yet the inflow will be retrograde through the lateral superior genicular vessels. Eventually, the lateral circumflex femoral vessels will be ligated to allow the flap to be elevated towards the distal thigh

The remainder of the skin can be elevated once the perforators are found. The proximal aspect of the descending branch of the LCFA is then ligated, which allows for the retrograde flow to the flap from the lateral superior genicular vessels. It is advisable to confirm flow in this vessel prior to the proximal ligation. Once the proximal pedicle is ligated, the flap can be elevated out of the muscle bed towards the distal thigh wound (Fig. 19.8).

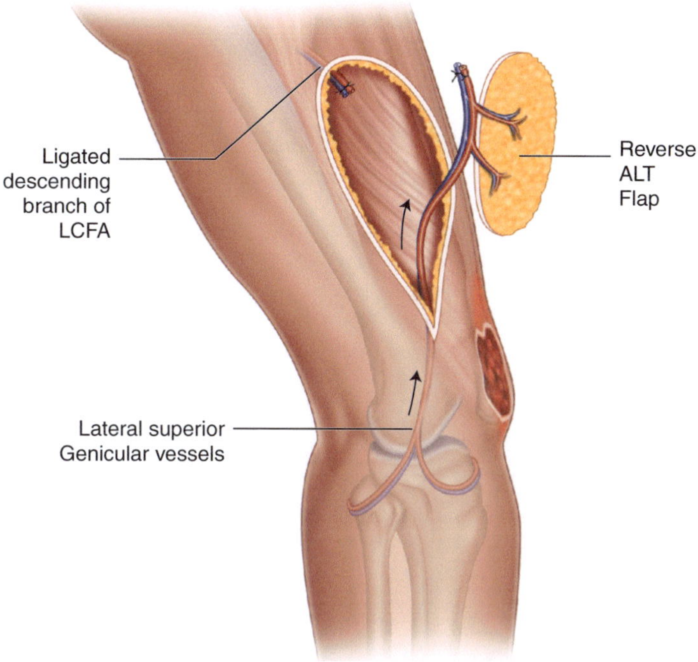

FIGURE 19.8 The reverse ALT flap has been elevated by selecting perforators from the descending branch of the lateral circumflex femoral vessels. The proximal pedicle has been ligated and divided; now the flap has retrograde flow from the lateral superior genicular vessels. The donor site wound may be connected to the primary wound to allow the flap to be inset

Wound Closure

Once the reverse ALT has been rotated into position, it may be sutured in place. The donor site is closed either primarily or with a split-thickness skin graft. A drain is usually placed in the region.

References

1. Acland RD, Schusterman M, Godina M, Eder E, Taylor GI, Carlisle I. The saphenous neurovascular free flap. Plast Reconstr Surg. 1981;67(6):763–74.
2. Pignatti M, Pasqualini M, Governa M, Bruti M, Rigotti G. Propeller flaps for leg reconstruction. J Plast Reconst Aesthet Surg. 2008;61(7):777–83.
3. Demirserena M, Efendioglua K, Demiralp C, Kılıçarslan K, Akkayaa H. Clinical experience with a reverse-flow anterolateral thigh perforator flap for the reconstruction of soft-tissue defects of the knee and proximal lower leg. J Plast Reconstr Aesthet Surg. 2011;64(12):1613–20.

Chapter 20
Soft Tissue Reconstruction for the Knee and Proximal Tibia

Victoria Wickenheisser, Benjamin Googe, and Scott T. Hollenbeck

Wounds in the knee region are very common, secondary to trauma or orthopedic procedures. When hardware is associated with the wound, flap coverage is often needed. Additionally, because the knee is a very flexible joint, secondary healing and skin grafting are seldom adequate primary options for wound closure.

V. Wickenheisser
Division of Plastic and Reconstructive Surgery, Duke University Hospital, Durham, NC, USA

B. Googe
Division of Plastic and Reconstructive Surgery, University of Mississippi Medical Center, Jackson, MS, USA

S. T. Hollenbeck (✉)
Division of Plastic and Reconstructive Surgery, Duke University Medical Center, Durham, NC, USA
e-mail: scott.hollenbeck@duke.edu

S. T. Hollenbeck et al. (eds.), *Handbook of Lower Extremity Reconstruction*, https://doi.org/10.1007/978-3-030-41035-3_20

Overview of the Gastrocnemius and Medial Sural Artery Perforator (mSAP) Flap

The gastrocnemius is a type I muscle flap; its vascular origins are the medial and lateral sural arteries. The muscle can be divided along its midline to generate either a medial or lateral muscle flap. The medial gastrocnemius is the most common variation of this muscle flap (Fig. 20.1). The lateral gastrocne-

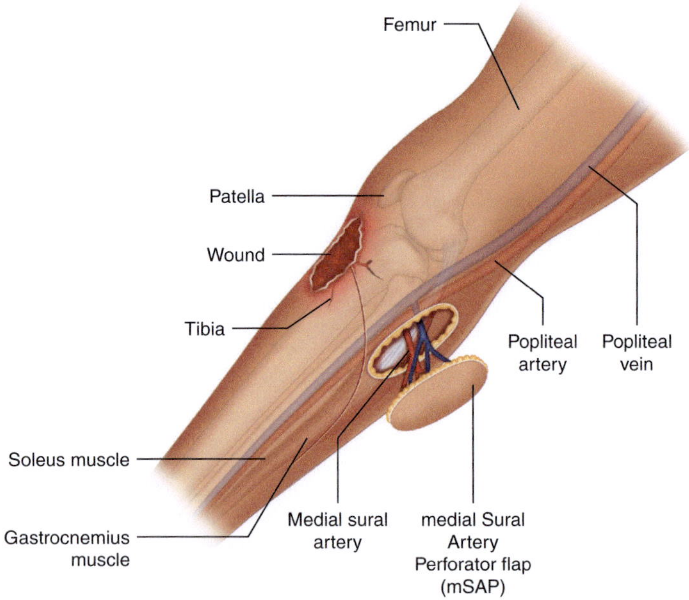

FIGURE 20.1 Medial gastrocnemius and medial sural artery perforator flap for lower knee coverage. The traumatic knee wound extends down to the level of the proximal tibia. The medial gastrocnemius muscle, which has blood supply from the medial sural artery, can be identified within the superficial aspect of the posterior calf. An incision can be extended from the anterior wound towards the posterior calf to allow for flap dissection and placement. The medial Sural Artery Perforator (mSAP) flap is positioned over a perforator that is exiting the gastrocnemius muscle

mius flap is less commonly used because it is somewhat limited in its arc of rotation, owing to the lateral head of the fibula and the common peroneal nerve. The gastrocnemius flap is typically performed as a muscle-only flap. The medial sural artery also supplies the skin of the posterior calf with blood through perforators extending through the gastrocnemius muscle. A perforator skin flap can be designed in this area and used for coverage of the anterior knee or proximal tibia [1].

Markings for the Gastrocnemius and mSAP Flap

The gastrocnemius muscle can be easily accessed by an incision along the posterior calf, but it is often advantageous to place the incision along the medial (or lateral) aspect of the posterior calf so that the muscle can be divided and more easily placed into the anterior knee region. The incision to access the gastrocnemius muscle may extend into the primary wound to allow the muscle to be laid easily into the defect. The mSAP flap is based on perforators extending through the gastrocnemius flap. A skin island can be designed around one of these perforators [2].

Gastrocnemius Flap Elevation

The medial gastrocnemius flap may be approached from a posterior and medial perspective. The median raphe of the muscle can be identified between the medial and lateral heads of the gastrocnemius muscle. The small saphenous vein and sural nerve usually run in this interval. The median raphe is split and the distal aspect of the muscle is split where it becomes mostly tendinous (Fig. 20.2). The deep surface of the medial head can be dissected off the soleus by blunt dissection proximally, but it must be sharply separated distally. This plane can be identified by the plantaris tendon. The pedicle of the flap is difficult to see unless the dissection extends into the popliteal fossa. The proximal origin of the muscle can also be divided in order to allow for additional length of rotation. It is also possible to increase the length

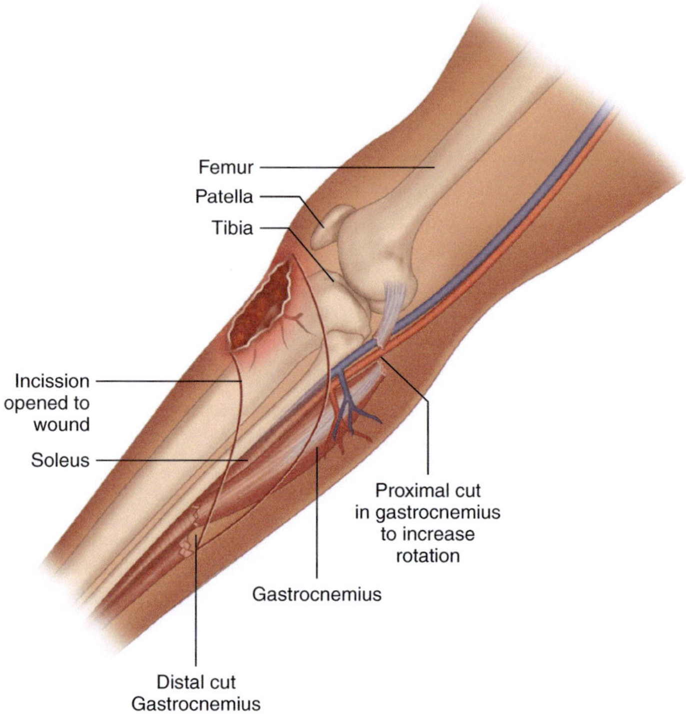

FIGURE 20.2 Dissection of the gastrocnemius flap. With the wound extended, the gastrocnemius muscle can be easily visualized with posterior traction. The muscle is divided along the median raphe and distally. The proximal aspect of the muscle may be divided above the pedicle to increase rotation

and width of the muscle by scoring the fascia of the muscle on the deep or superficial surfaces, or both.

Wound Closure

Once the gastrocnemius muscle has been rotated into position it may be sutured in place to adjacent connective tissue such that it lies directly over the tibial wound (Fig. 20.3). The skin defect may be partially closed. A skin graft may be placed over the muscle. A drain is usually placed in the

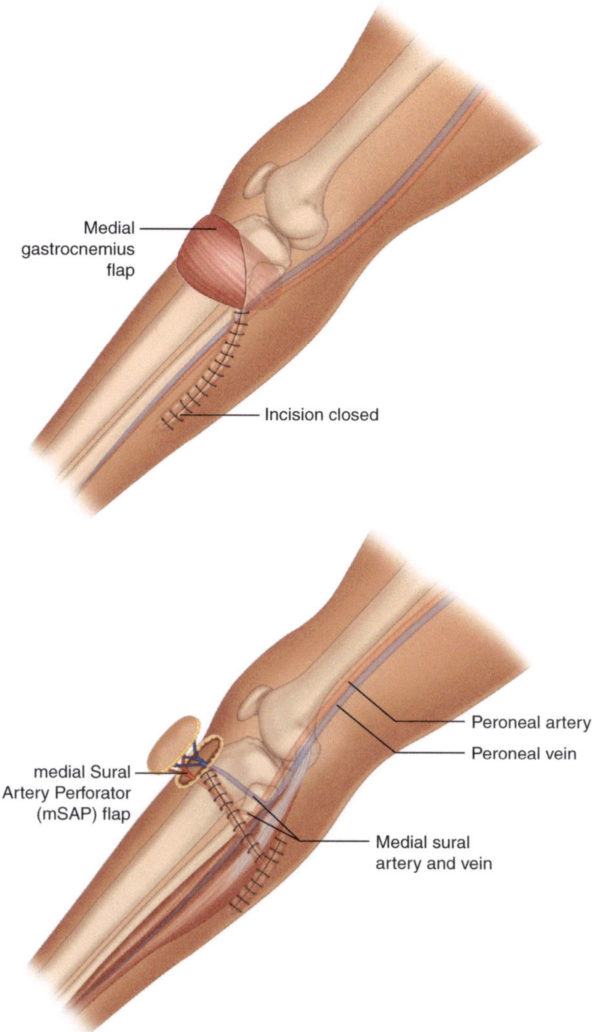

FIGURE 20.3 Closure of lower knee wound with a medial gastrocnemius or mSAP flap. The gastrocnemius muscle is placed over the anterior tibia, and a skin graft may then be performed (*top*). An mSAP flap is transferred to the anterior tibia after dissecting the pedicle out of the gastrocnemius muscle. The flap is either passed under the gastrocnemius muscle, or fibers of the muscle are split to allow the pedicle to extend directly to the wound (*bottom*)

region. The medial Sural Artery Perforator flap is positioned similarly to the gastrocnemius flap. The donor site is either closed primarily or with a split thickness skin graft.

References

1. Hallock G. Medial sural artery perforator free flap: legitimate use as a solution for the ipsilateral distal lower extremity defect. J Reconstr Microsurg. 2014;30(3):187–92.
2. McCraw J, Fishman J, Sharzer L. The versatile gastrocnemius myocutaneous flap. Plast Reconstr Surg. 1978;62(1):15–23.

Chapter 21
Soft Tissue Reconstruction of the Middle Third of the Tibia

Benjamin Googe, Somjade J. Songcharoen, and Peter B. Arnold

Wounds in the middle third of the tibia can occur after trauma. Coverage of exposed bone and hardware is paramount for extremity salvage. Skin and subcutaneous fat overlying the anterior tibial surface is very thin, and wounds presenting in this area can be challenging for primary closure due to paucity of soft tissue. Soleus and tibialis anterior pedicled muscle flaps provide the bulk of local reconstructive options for durable autologous soft tissue coverage in this area [1–4] (Fig. 21.1).

B. Googe · S. J. Songcharoen · P. B. Arnold (✉)
Division of Plastic and Reconstructive Surgery, University of Mississippi Medical Center, Jackson, MS, USA
e-mail: parnold@umc.edu

S. T. Hollenbeck et al. (eds.), *Handbook of Lower Extremity Reconstruction*, https://doi.org/10.1007/978-3-030-41035-3_21

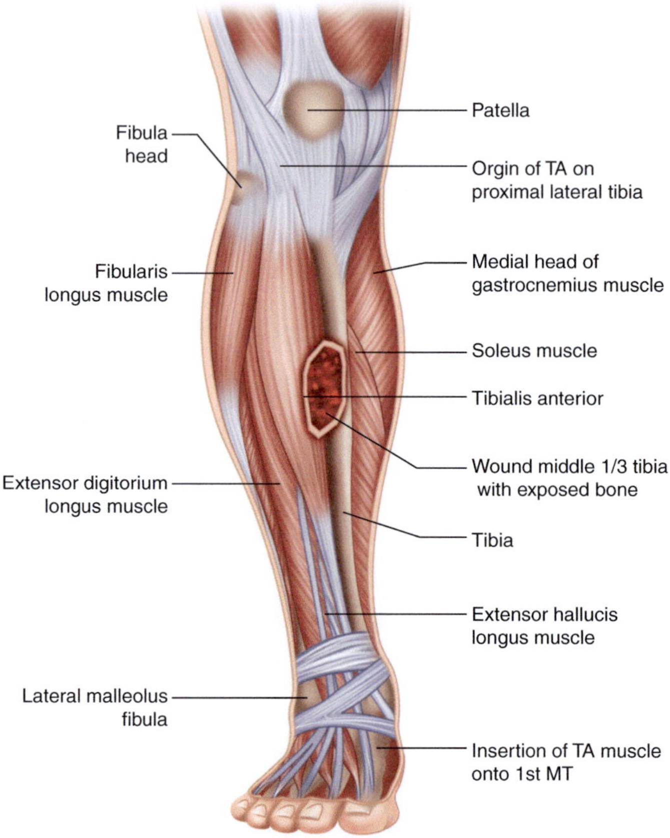

FIGURE 21.1 Middle-third tibia wound, with exposed bone. Local options for this wound include a soleus flap from the superficial posterior compartment, or a flap using the tibialis anterior (TA) muscle, which lies in the anterior compartment directly adjacent to the wound, along the surface of the tibia. MT—metatarsal

Soleus Flap

The soleus flap, a Mathes and Nahai type II flap, is a bipennate muscle flap running the length of the lower leg in the superficial posterior compartment, just deep to the gastrocnemius. It receives dominant arterial pedicles from the popliteal artery, proximal two posterior tibial branches, and proximal two peroneal branches, and minor contributions from the distal three or four segmental branches of the posterior tibial artery [4–6]. The muscle originates from a tendinous arch between the tibia and fibula heads as well as proximal posterior aspects of the tibia and fibula shafts [7]. Distally, the soleus (with other superficial posterior compartment muscles) inserts onto the posterior calcaneus as the Achilles tendon [7] (Fig. 21.2). The flap can be split as a hemisoleus flap or rotated for a distally based reversed soleus flap, depending on the size of the defect and requirements for reconstruction [8, 9]. It has been utilized from the distal knee at the lower margin of gastrocnemius flap coverage to the distal third of the lower leg when based distally from the inferior perforators, but its most reliable and traditional indication is for soft tissue coverage of the middle third of the distal leg [5, 8, 9].

Markings for the Soleus Flap

The incision can be placed axially on the medial or lateral aspects, depending on the anticipated arc of rotation. For most indications, a medially based flap is preferred, as the dissection is easier and there is more forgiveness in the amount of soft tissue for local rearrangement once the flap is rotated into place. For a medially based soleus flap for mid-tibial coverage, skin markings and the subsequent initial incision will begin on the medial lower leg at the level of the tibial plateau and will be carried distally to 2–3 cm proximal to the medial malleolus [8].

Soleus Flap Elevation

When possible, a tourniquet should be placed on the thigh and inflated to allow for a bloodless dissection. For a medially based soleus flap, elevation is based on identifying and preserving perforators from the posterior tibial artery entering the muscle belly deep surface. The incision is made in the medial aspect of the leg from the tibial plateau to just proximal to the medial

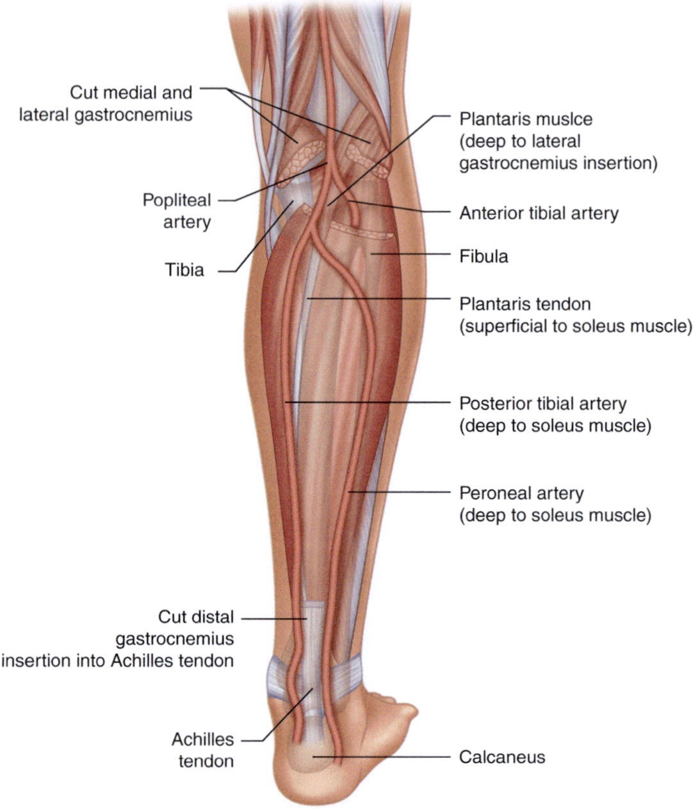

FIGURE 21.2 Soleus flap for middle third tibia coverage. The soleus flap is designed based on perforators off the popliteal, posterior tibial, and peroneal arteries, depending on how the muscle is rotated. When rotated medially, perforators entering on the deep surface of the muscle will be encountered, arising from the posterior tibial artery in the deep posterior compartment. Distal perforators may need to be ligated to obtain a good arc of rotation

malleolus. The superficial posterior compartment can be identified by finding the plane between the gastrocnemius and the soleus, with the plantaris between as an identifiable landmark. The soleus is elevated starting in the middle and proceeding proximally and distally. Once the plane is identified, the muscle can be dissected rapidly and freed from its superficial surface by passing a hand between it and the overlying gastrocnemius. The deep surface dissection is more tedious, as the neurovascular bundles of the deep posterior compartment and the perforators of the flap enter in this plane. The most distal extent of the flap can be released from the Achilles tendon and the flap retracted medially. Perforators from the posterior tibial artery will need to be ligated in a distal-to-proximal fashion to free the muscle until enough length is mobilized for rotation into the defect anteriorly (Fig. 21.3). To minimize the number of perforators that require ligation, care must be taken to dissect proximally as little as necessary to gain the desired length; fewer than half of patients have a direct branch of the popliteal artery to the soleus [10]. For smaller defects, dividing the soleus longitudinally along its raphe can allow for more mobility and minimize donor site morbidity.

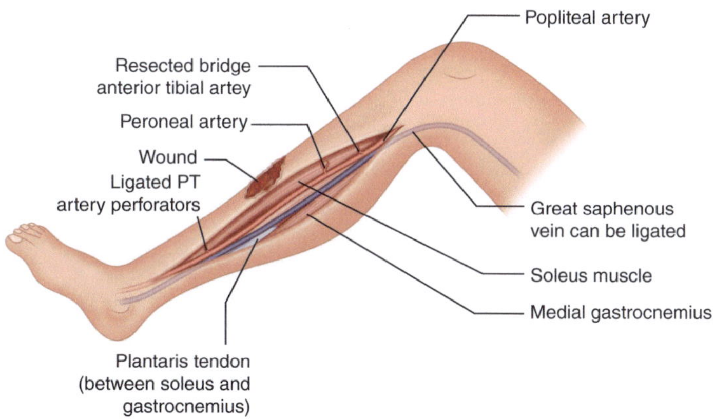

Figure 21.3 Elevation of the soleus flap. Marking and incision are made in the medial aspect of the leg from the tibial plateau to just proximal to the medial malleolus. The superficial posterior compartment can be identified by finding the plane between the gastrocnemius and the soleus, with the plantaris between as an identifiable landmark. The soleus is elevated starting in the middle. Distal perforators from the posterior tibial (PT) artery are ligated to provide for arc of rotation. The great saphenous vein may need to be ligated, and small skin bridges between wound and incision, excised

Wound Closure

The donor defect can generally be closed primarily, as the flap is generally harvested without an overlying skin paddle unless a gastrocnemius flap is used concurrently. A drain should be left in this dead space and pulled when output has decreased appropriately. Tissue rearrangement on the medial aspect of the leg is forgiving and can be reorganized around the muscle pedicle. Small skin bridges between the muscle and wound should be excised, as an already tenuous blood supply will be further compromised. Definitive coverage of the soleus muscle will require skin grafting over the flap. This can be placed at time of the flap, or it can be delayed if the blood supply to the flap is questionable. A knee immobilizer should be placed at the conclusion of the procedure to minimize undue tension on the flap's closure.

Tibialis Anterior Flap

The tibialis anterior flap, a Mathes and Nahai type IV flap, uses the muscle located in the anterior compartment adjacent to and along the lateral aspect of the tibia, with a vascular supply based on segmental perforators from the anterior tibial artery. It is best utilized for narrow, longitudinally oriented wounds on the anterior surface of the tibia. To minimize donor morbidity, the muscle is most commonly splint longitudinally to preserve maximal function of ankle dorsiflexion [1–3].

Markings for the Tibialis Anterior Flap

Two variations of the flap can be utilized for coverage, a proximally based transposition flap or a turnover flap. Both have similar markings and initial dissection. A longitudinal marking is made just lateral to the wound on the anterior surface of tibia, and extended proximally and distally along the lateral margin of the wound to allow for increased exposure if needed.

Elevation of the Tibialis Anterior Flap

An incision is made in the region of the previous marking at the level of the wound and extended proximally and distally until sufficient length of the tibialis anterior is accessible for adequate wound coverage. The fascia overlying the muscle is divided longitudinally on its most lateral surface to allow for lateral dissection around the muscle, to gain exposure to its deep surface. The deep surface can be elevated and dissected to identify and preserve perforators from the anterior tibial artery (Fig. 21.4). Starting at the level of the wound, the muscle can then be divided longitudinally distally and proximally to slide the muscle over the wound under a minimal amount of tension. Care must be taken to avoid injury to perforators. Once sufficiently mobilized, the flap can be sutured to the edge of the defect to hold its position.

Alternatively, the muscle can be utilized as a turnover flap. The initial dissection is similar, but rather than incising the

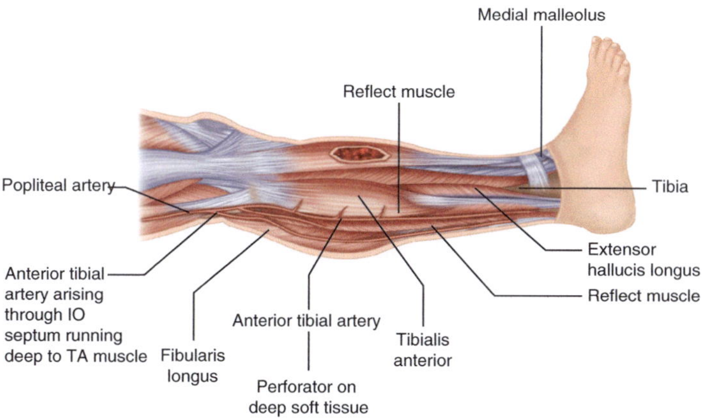

Figure 21.4 Tibialis anterior flap. The tibialis anterior (TA) muscle can be elevated based on deep perforators from the anterior tibial artery. Dividing the muscle longitudinally on the lateral surface proximally and distally from the level of the wound can provide release to slide muscle over the wound with minimal tension. Alternatively, a turnover flap can be utilized. IO—interosseous

muscle longitudinally, dissection is carried on from lateral to medial along the deep surface of the flap, to allow the muscle to transpose over itself, flipping along the axis of its medial attachment. Dissection must be sufficient proximally and distally so as to avoid undue tension on the perforators as they rotate over and become superficial along the flap's surface after it is flipped into the wound bed. Longitudinal incision on the deep surface can decrease the amount of tension on the flap prior to inset.

Wound Closure

Once the tibialis anterior flap has been advanced over the exposed bone, a skin graft can be placed over the flap and resulting donor site defect. This can be performed at the sentinel operation or can be delayed if flap perfusion is deemed tenuous. Strict limitation of ankle motion should be maintained with an ankle-foot orthosis or boot to prevent tension on the flap following closure.

References

1. Panse N, Sahasrabudhe P, Pande G, Chandanwale A, Dhongde R, Rajpal L. The split tibialis anterior muscle flap - a simple solution for longitudinal middle third tibial defects. Indian J Plast Surg. 2012;45:53–7. https://doi.org/10.4103/0970-0358.96585.
2. Li X, Yang ZP, Li JM. Soft tissue reconstruction with sagittal split anterior tibial muscle transfer and medial gastrocnemius transposition in limb-salvage surgery of bone tumors in a proximal tibia. Ann Plast Surg. 2008;61:204–8. https://doi.org/10.1097/SAP.0b013e318157dae7.
3. Hallock GG. Sagittal split tibialis anterior muscle flap. Ann Plast Surg. 2002;49:39–43.
4. Gravvanis A, Kyriakopoulos A, Kateros K, Tsoutsos D. Flap reconstruction of the knee: a review of current concepts and a proposed algorithm. World J Orthop. 2014;5:603–13. https://doi.org/10.5312/wjo.v5.i5.603.

5. Hyodo I, Nakayama B, Takahashi M, Toriyama K, Kamei Y, Torii S. The gastrocnemius with soleus bi-muscle flap. Br J Plast Surg. 2004;57:77–82.
6. Mathes SJ, Nahai F. Vascular anatomy of muscle: classification and application. In: Mathes SJ, Nahai F, editors. Clinical applications for muscle and musculocutaneous flaps. St. Louis: CV Mosby; 1982. p. 16–94.
7. Drake R, Vogl AW, Mitchell A. Gray's anatomy for students. 4th ed. Philadelphia: Elsevier; 2019.
8. Strauch B, Vasconez LO, Hall-Findlay EJ, Lee BT. Grabb's encyclopedia of flaps. 3rd ed. Philadelphia: Lippincott Williams & Wilkins; 2009.
9. Pu LL. Successful soft-tissue coverage of a tibial wound in the distal third of the leg with a medial hemisoleus muscle flap. Plast Reconstr Surg. 2005;115:245–51.
10. Prathapamchandra V, Prabhu LV, Pai MM, Murlimanju BV, Vadgaonkar R. Arterial supply to the soleus muscle: an anatomical study with emphasis on its application in the pedicle flap surgery. Surg Radiol Anat. 2015;37:1055–61. https://doi.org/10.1007/s00276-015-1485-9.

Chapter 22
Soft Tissue Reconstruction of the Distal Third Tibia

Benjamin Googe, Somjade J. Songcharoen, and Peter B. Arnold

Wounds in the distal third of the tibia can be considered the most challenging for reconstruction and lower extremity salvage. This "no man's land" provides very limited local reconstructive options because of its paucity of soft tissue laxity and redundancy. To this end, most reconstructive surgeons view distal-third injuries as requiring free tissue transfer for adequate soft tissue reconstruction. In limited circumstances, however, there are several viable options for local, pedicled soft tissue reconstruction in the distal third. These include the reverse sural artery flap, bipedicled flaps, propeller perforator flaps, and keystone flaps.

When attempting any locally based flaps in the distal third of the lower extremity, it is critical for the surgeon to consider the concept of zone of injury, especially in the traumatized extremity. Although any particular soft tissue deficit may be small, the area affected by the injury is often quite large. When the pedicle of a flap is within this zone of injury, flow into and out of the flap can be negatively affected (Fig. 22.1) [1].

B. Googe · S. J. Songcharoen · P. B. Arnold (✉)
Division of Plastic and Reconstructive Surgery, University of Mississippi Medical Center, Jackson, MS, USA
e-mail: parnold@umc.edu

S. T. Hollenbeck et al. (eds.), *Handbook of Lower Extremity Reconstruction*, https://doi.org/10.1007/978-3-030-41035-3_22

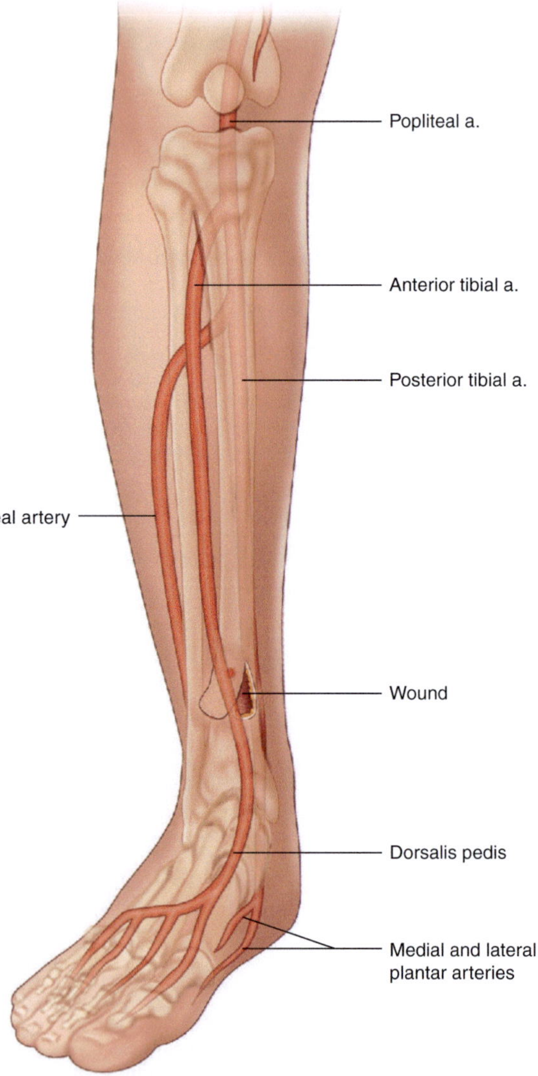

FIGURE 22.1 Distal third tibia wound. There is a wound in the distal third of the tibia with exposed bone. Local options are limited but include the reverse sural artery perforator flap and local tissue transposition flaps. Blood supply will depend on perforators from the underlying vasculature

Overview of the Reverse Sural Artery Flap

The reverse sural flap is a distally based fasciocutaneous flap based on recurrent flow *from perforators off the peroneal artery at the level of the ankle.* The paddle of the flap originates on the posterior aspect of the leg, midway between the knee and ankle; its pedicle runs down the central leg and then tails toward the lateral malleolus. This flap is best used for small to mid-size defects in the distal third of the lower leg and when there is little concern for ancillary trauma to the ankle or peroneal artery, which may compromise blood flow to the flap. The flap is harvested in a suprafascial or subfascial plane; most surgeons opt to harvest the fascia with the flap, believing that doing so will potentially improve perfusion.

Markings for the Reverse Sural Flap

When used for distal third tibia defects, markings can be made on the posterior leg along the axis of the sural nerve, with the skin island placed midway between the knee and ankle. The tail of the pedicle will migrate towards the lateral malleolus about 5 cm above the ankle, to allow a pivot point that incorporates perforators from the peroneal artery (Fig. 22.2).

Reverse Sural Flap Elevation

The reverse sural flap can be an island based on an adipofascial pedicle (Fig. 22.3) to allow for primary closure of the donor site, or it can be elevated full-thickness in a fasciocutaneous manner. The skin island is elevated full-thickness, including fascia, down to the gastrocnemius muscle. An adipofascial pedicle 2–4 cm wide is elevated along the axis of (and including) the sural artery, smaller saphenous vein, and sural nerve distally until a point about 5 cm above the lateral malleolus, which will be the pivot point as the entry point of a peroneal artery perforator [2].

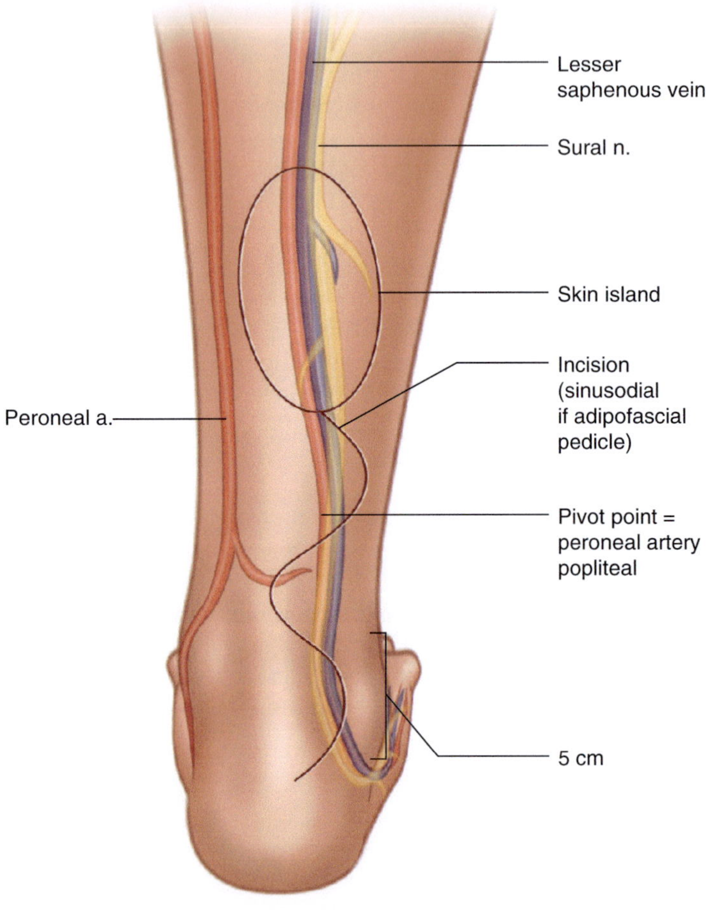

FIGURE 22.2 Reverse sural flap for distal third tibia coverage. The reverse sural (rSural) flap is distally based and supplied by perforators from the peroneal artery. Marking for the skin island is midway between the knee and ankle and centered on the posterior aspect of the lower leg. The pedicle pivots around the perforators, which enter the pedicle about 5 cm above the lateral malleolus

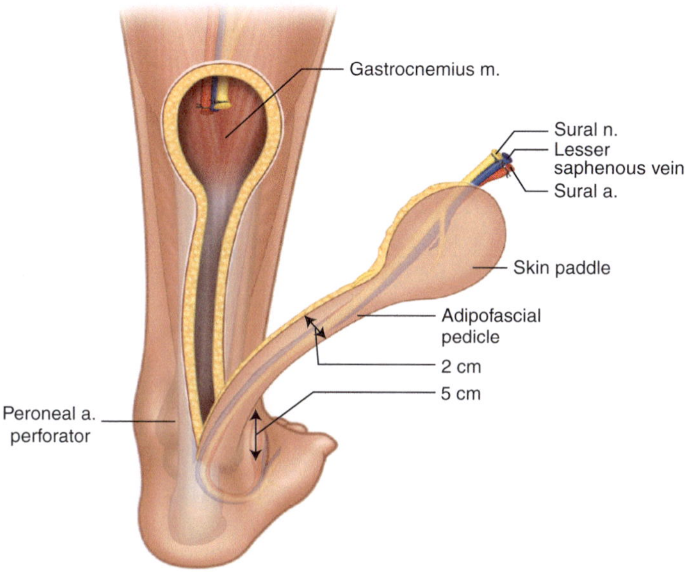

FIGURE 22.3 Elevation of reverse sural flap. The sinusoidal incision is opened though the dermis along the axis of the sural artery, smaller saphenous vein, and sural nerve. The skin island is incised and elevated down to the gastrocnemius muscle. The flap is elevated proximally to distally, incorporating a 2-cm-wide adipofascial flap around the neurovascular structures to the pivot point 5 cm above the lateral malleolus

Wound Closure

The skin island site will most commonly be closed with a split-thickness skin graft placed over the gastrocnemius muscle. The skin overlying the pedicle can be closed primarily if an adipofascial pedicle is used. If a fasciocutaneous pedicle is used, a skin graft may be needed.

Overview of Local Transposition and Rotational Flaps

For smaller defects when free tissue transfer is a less attractive option, local flaps can provide a suitable alternative. Bipedicle, propeller, and keystone flaps are among the most frequently utilized. Blood supply to these flaps can be random or can use a perforator from a named vessel near the defect. Judicious use of these flaps can preclude more complex reconstructive options for extremity salvage.

Bipedicled Flap

Bipedicled fasciocutaneous flaps, based on a random axis blood supply from two pedicles, and was originally described as an alternative to the cross-leg flap [3]. These flaps are best for smaller defects (<5 cm) in the lower leg, though use of double flaps can increase their utility. The flap is taken from the longitudinal side of the defect and is approximately 5 cm in width. The flap is usually 2–3 cm longer than the wound on each side, to allow for advancement under minimal tension. Blood supply comes from the proximal and distal attachments.

The use of bipedicled flaps should be considered for smaller wounds in patients who are not candidates for advanced reconstructive procedures, where there is limited orthopaedic hardware exposure, and where it is anticipated that the amount of surrounding soft tissue damage is limited. The donor sites are acceptable, and the tissue match is usually superior to any other reconstructive option, but one must expect a relatively high rate of postoperative complications, which can include partial flap necrosis, dehiscence, and cellulitis (Fig. 22.4) [4].

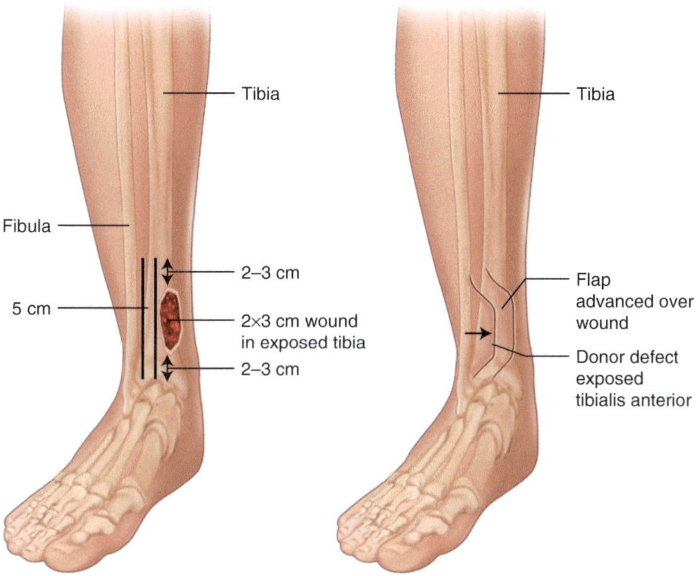

FIGURE 22.4 The bipedicled flap can be used to cover a wound over the distal tibia with exposed bone. The flap, about 5 cm in width, lies along the lateral aspect of the wound and is 2–3 cm longer on the proximal and distal ends to allow for advancement. The flap is elevated down to fascia overlying the tibialis anterior muscle

Propeller Flap

The propeller flap has emerged as a powerful tool in extremity reconstruction owing to its relative ease of elevation and the ability to move a relatively large amount of tissue locally. This method of soft tissue reconstruction does not require disruption of axial vessels or muscle, making it an ideal donor tissue. Additionally, like all local flaps in the distal third of the lower extremity, tissue match is close to ideal [5].

Flap design involves the identification of several possible fasciocutaneous perforator vessels that are able to provide nourishing flow to the tissue planned to be moved. Perforators off of any of the three named arteries in the lower third are acceptable. Identification is most often accomplished by preoperative imaging and with hand-held Doppler probes during the procedure. Once suitable vessels are identified, the flap is elevated, typically in the subfascial plane, and the perforating vessel is directly visualized. If the caliber and condition of the vessel are deemed suitable, the remainder of the flap is elevated. Once the flap is isolated on the pedicle, the vessels are typically dissected down towards the main pedicle to allow for rotation of the flap. It is possible to rotate these flaps 180 degrees under most circumstances (Fig. 22.5). An expected

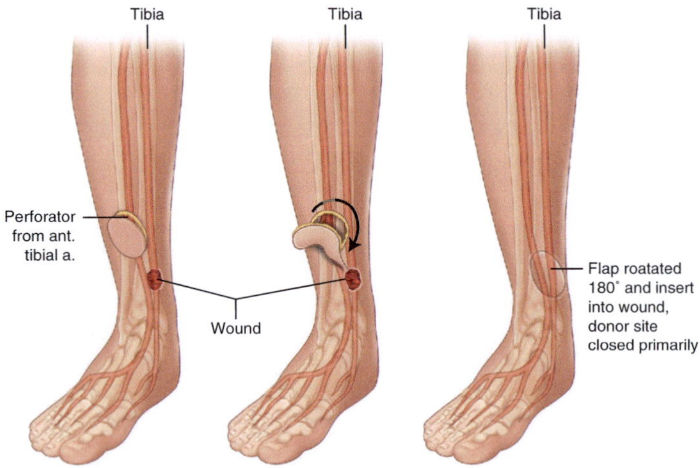

FIGURE 22.5 The propeller flap is based on a perforator from the anterior tibial artery. The skin island lies over the tibialis anterior muscle. After rotating 180 degrees, the donor site can be closed primarily (as depicted) or with a skin graft

complication rate of 14% should be considered, especially in areas where partial flap loss will involve exposure of underlying structures such as bone, tendon, and hardware [4].

Keystone Flap

The keystone flap, a local fasciocutaneous flap based along the longitudinal aspect of the wound, is based on the underlying known perforators present within the flap. It is typically used when there is a small defect and minimal compromise of surrounding soft tissue. Flaps can be designed alongside any aspect of the defect, but ideally they should be placed parallel to known perforators, to increase the chance of incorporating these vessels within the flap [5].

If possible, flaps should be designed to be larger than the defect, in order to recruit as many perforators as possible. The flap is incised through the level of the fascia, and minimal undermining is carried out towards the central portion of the flap, taking care to preserve as many arteries and veins as possible (Fig. 22.6). The corners of the donor site are closed in a V-Y fashion to aid in advancement and closure of the donor site primarily, which can be accomplished in 85% of cases [6]. One must be aware that the limited laxity of the soft tissues of the lower third of the tibia limits the utilization of the keystone flap to close large defects.

Wound Closure

Once the flaps have been advanced over exposed vital structures, the donor site can be closed primarily, or a skin graft can be applied.

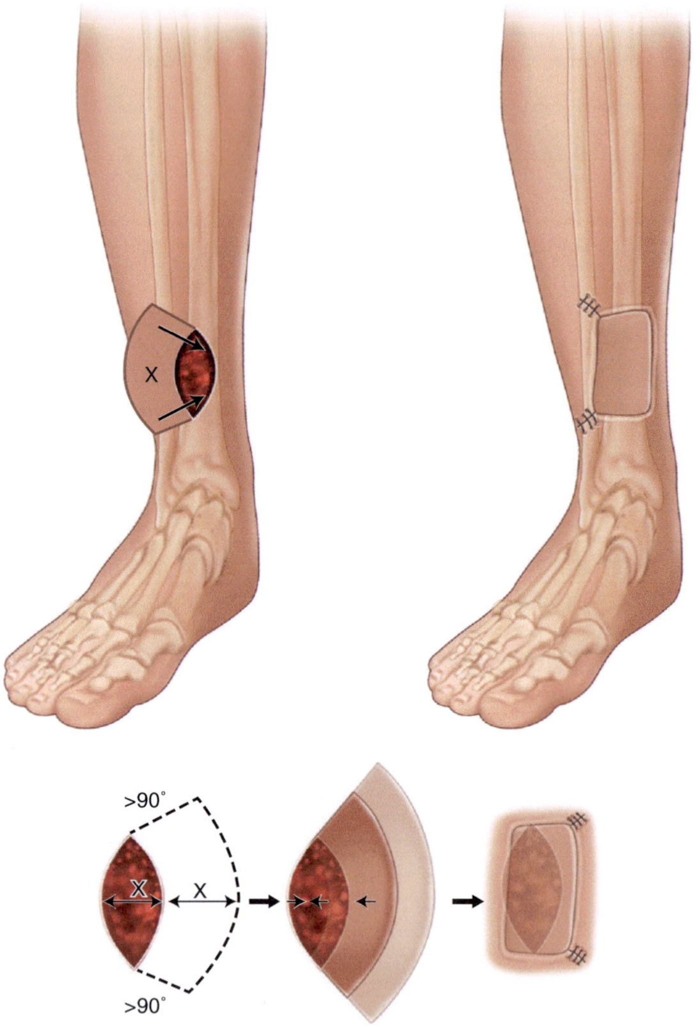

FIGURE 22.6 The keystone flap. On the left are seen the preoperative markings, with final transposition and inset on the right. The diagrams below show enlarged markings and transposition of the flap. Note that the defect is the same width as the flap, but the flap is longer longitudinally than the wound, with approximately a 90-degree angle at the proximal and distal aspects. As the flap is advanced, the corners of the donor site are closed in a V-Y fashion

References

1. Kolker AR, Kasabian AK, Karp NS, Gottlieb JJ. Fate of free flap microanastomosis distal to the zone of injury in lower extremity trauma. Plast Reconstr Surg. 1997;99:1068–73.
2. Sugg KB, Schaub TA, Concannon MJ, Cederna PS, Brown DL. The reverse superficial sural artery flap revisited for complex lower extremity and foot reconstruction. Plast Reconstr Surg Glob Open. 2015;3:e519.
3. Crawford. Cross-leg flap repairs. Ann R Coll Surg Engl. 1981;63(1):63.
4. Granzow JW, Ki A, Suliman A, Caton A, Goldberg M, Boyd JB. Bipedicled flaps in posttraumatic lower extremity reconstruction. J Plast Reconstr Aesthet Surg. 2013;66:1415–20.
5. Mendieta M, Cabrerea R, Sui A, Altamirano R, Gutierrez S. Perforator propeller flaps for the coverage of middle and distal leg soft-tissue defects. Plast Reconstr Surg Glob Open. 2018;6:e1759.
6. Gomez OJ, Baron OR, Penarredonda ML. Keystone flap: overcoming paradigms. Plast Reconstr Surg Glob Open. 2019;7:e2126.

Chapter 23
Soft Tissue Reconstruction of the Foot

Benjamin Googe, Somjade J. Songcharoen, and Peter B. Arnold

The successful soft tissue reconstruction of the foot requires a comprehensive multidisciplinary team. Wounds of the feet stem from a multitude of problems, including physical defects from trauma and tumor resection, medical conditions such as diabetes and peripheral vascular disease, and congenital anomalies including structural, gait, and vascular abnormalities. Thus, many specialties must be involved, including foot and ankle orthopedics, vascular surgery, plastic and reconstructive surgery, oncology, endocrinology, infectious disease, physical and occupational therapy, prosthetics, and social work. Successful reconstruction of foot wounds requires not only durable soft tissue coverage but also interventions to prevent recurrence. This chapter focuses on local flaps and their utility in reconstructing common wounds of the foot.

B. Googe · S. J. Songcharoen · P. B. Arnold (✉)
Division of Plastic and Reconstructive Surgery,
University of Mississippi Medical Center, Jackson, MS, USA
e-mail: parnold@umc.edu

S. T. Hollenbeck et al. (eds.), *Handbook of Lower Extremity Reconstruction*, https://doi.org/10.1007/978-3-030-41035-3_23

Dorsal Wounds

The soft tissue of the dorsum of the foot is thin and pliable. It overlies the extensor tendon mechanism, which undergoes a significant amount of excursion with gliding of the tendons. Local flaps are thus well suited for reconstruction of defects, offering durable coverage coupled with pliability and contour necessary to accept footwear or prosthetics. These flaps depend on adequate blood supply related to the dorsalis pedis artery.

Dorsalis Pedis Flap

The dorsalis pedis flap (Fig. 23.1) is a thin, dorsally based flap that can be raised as an axial, pedicled fasciocutaneous or myocutaneous flap. It has been used to successfully cover wounds of the medial and lateral malleoli, Achilles tendon, heel, and the distal third of the tibia [1].

Markings for the Dorsalis Pedis Flap

The dorsalis pedis artery may be palpated at the dorsum of the ankle. A line drawn from this point to the first webspace marks the long axis of the flap. The flap is then designed symmetrically along this axis. The proximal border should be distal to the extensor retinaculum [1] and the distal extent should be proximal to the tarsometaphalangeal joint [2]. Transversely, the flap may extend from the tendon of the extensor hallucis longus to the extensor digitorum longus [2] of the 5th toe. In the average adult foot, a flap can be raised measuring 12 × 9 cm [1].

Dorsalis Pedis Flap Elevation

Flap elevation occurs under a bloodless field using a tourniquet. The distal incision is made at the first web space, and

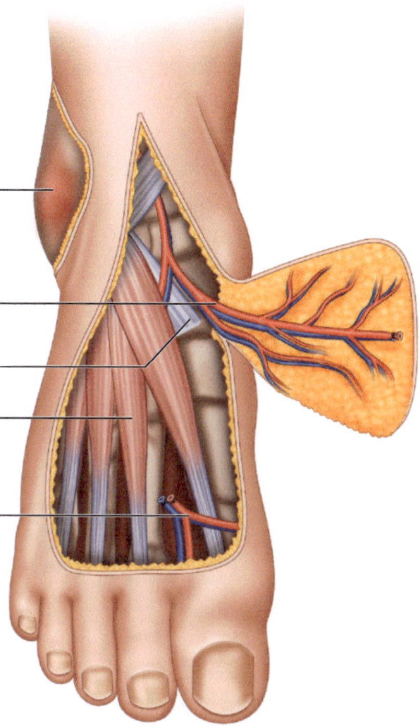

FIGURE 23.1 Dorsalis pedis flap. A dorsal view of the foot with a fasciocutaneous island flap based proximally on the dorsalis pedis artery and venae comitantes. The artery has been tied off at the junction of the first metatarsal artery. In this picture, the cruciate crural ligament has been cut to allow pedicle rotation. A lateral ankle wound is shown as a possible coverage option

the first dorsal metatarsal artery is identified, ligated, and divided. Dissection continues from distal to proximal and medial to lateral. The superficial peroneal nerve may be preserved as a part of the flap or excluded in the dissection. The plane of dissection occurs deep to the first dorsal metatarsal artery but preserves the paratenon of the extensor tendons. As originally described, two layers of fascia cover the extensor hallucis longus tendon: a thick superficial fascia and a more delicate, deep muscular fascia. Both must be raised to gain access to the bared surface of the second dorsal interosseus muscle. Care must be taken in the dissection of the distal dorsalis pedis artery, which is attached to the undersurface of the superficial fascia and constitutes the sole blood supply of the distal 3 cm of the flap [3]. More proximally, the dissection is kept close to the periosteum of the cuneiform bones [1]. Once the proximal incision is completed, the extensor retinaculum is opened to release the dorsalis pedis artery along with its venae comitantes and nerves. The extensor digitorum longus is retracted laterally, thereby exposing the underlying extensor digitorum brevis. The first head of the muscle may be taken as a part of the flap to preserve collateral blood supply to the flap. Once elevated, the lateral tarsal artery is then exposed coursing under the flexor digitorum brevis. This is then ligated and divided. The flap can now be isolated on the vascular pedicle. More proximal dissection can be undertaken to extend the length of the pedicle. The average length of the pedicle can be as long as 18 cm [2]. During inset, if a subcutaneous tunnel is chosen, care must be taken to avoid compression on bony prominences.

Alternatively, a distally based flap has been described [4]. The flap dissection progresses from proximal to distal, starting with identification of the dorsalis pedis artery. Anatomic variations have been described in which branches of the first metatarsal artery do not anastomose with the plantar arterial network. Therefore, the dorsalis pedis artery should not be ligated until adequate reverse flow is verified. This may be accomplished by clamping the dorsalis pedis once the flap is islanded [5]. The dissection continues, exposing the deep plantar branch and then the communicating branch between the first dorsal metatarsal artery and the plantar artery [4].

Wound Closure

If the extensor retinaculum was divided, it should be repaired to prevent bowstringing. After meticulous hemostasis, any defect in the tenosynovium should also be repaired. A split-thickness skin graft may be harvested with care to provide adequate tissue for the depths of the first interspace. Finally, a bolster dressing and splint should be placed in a way that will allow for flap monitoring [1].

Wounds of the Heel

Wounds of the weight-bearing areas of the foot present a reconstructive challenge in the contour and demands for durable, sensate, and specialized glabrous tissue. Although local options are fairly limited, they remain powerful tools in the armamentarium of the reconstructive surgeon.

Medial Plantar Flap

The medial plantar artery is indicated for reconstruction of local defects involving distal weight-bearing areas of the foot. It provides durable, sensate, glabrous skin from the instep of the foot with shock-absorbing fibrofatty subcutaneous tissue and plantar fascia [6], thus providing an ideal replacement of tissue using the so-called “like-with-like” premise. As such, the medial plantar artery flap (Fig. 23.2) is indicated for coverage of defects of the lateral sole and heel, as well as the lower Achilles [7].

Markings for the Medial Plantar Flap

The instep area of the foot extends from the navicular tuberosity on the medial border of the foot to the midline of the plantar surface. Proximally, it extends distal to the weight-bearing heel to a space just proximal to first metatarsal head [8]. A doppler probe may be used to find the posterior tibial artery and its bifurcation to the medial and lateral plantar arteries. Although the medial plantar artery will inevitably be located towards the medial border of larger flaps, distal perfusion is usually not affected. Care should be taken to

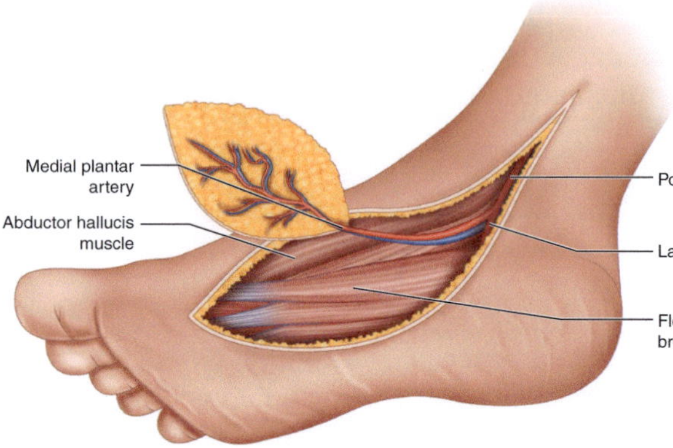

FIGURE 23.2 Medial plantar flap. This plantar view of the foot shows a fasciocutaneous flap based proximally on the medial plantar artery. Its course between the abductor hallucis and flexor digitorum brevis muscles is shown. Also shown is its bifurcation from the posterior tibial and lateral plantar artery. A medial malleolus defect can be a coverage option

keep the distal edge of the flap 2 cm proximal to the head of the first metatarsal [9]. A flap 10 cm long × 7 cm wide may be elevated without encroaching on the weight-bearing surface [10].

Medial Plantar Flap Elevation

Elevation begins at the medial margin of the proposed flap, which is incised and deepened through the fascia onto the abductor hallucis muscle. A subfascial dissection proceeds until the septum between the abductor hallucis and the flexor digitorum brevis is encountered. Several perforators of the medial plantar vessel can be identified through the intermuscular septum. Perforators are 0.3 mm, with smaller concomitant veins, so care must be taken to preserve the septum and surrounding adipose tissue around the perforator [11]. Here, dissection is deepened while preserving the septum. The abductor hallucis muscle is retracted medially to visualize the neurovascular bundle. Proximally, the division of the posterior tibial vessels is identified. The incision may then be extended proximally towards the posterior inferior margin of the medial malleolus. The origin of the abductor hallucis and its vascular branches must be divided, thereby exposing a pedicle 4–5 cm in length. Here the medial plantar nerve is identified, and lateral branches to the flap may be preserved. The distal margin of the flap is then incised. Slips of the plantar aponeurosis are cut, taking care not to injure the common digital nerve trunks to the toes. Finally, the lateral margin is incised along with the plantar aponeurosis. Again, dissection proceeds medially in the subfascial plane above the flexor digitorum brevis muscle until the medial aspect of the intermuscular septum is encountered. The proximal attachment of the plantar aponeurosis is divided, and the flap can then be transposed [9].

Flexor Digitorum Brevis Flap

The flexor digitorum brevis flap is indicated for small, deep defects of the plantar heel [12]. As a pedicled island flap, it can be used to resurface the medial and lateral malleoli in addition to the entire surface of the posterior superior aspect of the heel pad [13] (Fig. 23.3). Further, it can be sensate as a myocutaneous flap, via branches of the medial plantar nerve. A reverse-flow flap can also be accomplished with an intact distal plantar arch to cover distal foot defects in a pedicled fashion or as a V-Y advancement flap, gaining 2–3 cm [14].

Markings for the Flexor Digitorum Brevis Flap

The flexor digitorum brevis muscle originates on the medial process of the calcaneus, plantar aponeurosis, and intermuscular septum. It is located between the abductor hallucis and abductor digiti minimi, forming the first layer of muscles in the sole, just deep to the plantar aponeurosis. Deep to the muscle lies the flexor digitorum longus and

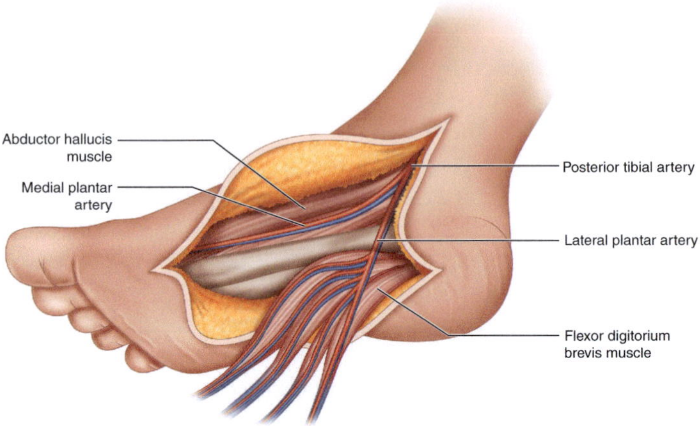

FIGURE 23.3 Flexor digitorum brevis flap. This plantar view shows the lateral plantar artery taking off from the medial plantar artery and the posterior tibial artery. The medial plantar artery runs medial to the abductor hallucis muscle. The skin is incised and retracted to reveal the flexor digitorum brevis muscle disinserted and turning over, with its pedicle running along the dorsal surface. A heel wound with exposed calcaneus can be a coverage option

quadratus plantae [15]. It has insertions to the middle phalanges of the 2nd to 5th toes. As a muscle-only flap, a linear incision can be drawn along the length of the third metatarsal for exposure. A doppler probe is useful for locating major and minor pedicles, to guide the design of an overlying skin paddle.

Flexor Digitorum Brevis Flap Elevation

A midline incision is used to expose the muscle, and dissection is carried through the skin and plantar fascia. The skin and plantar fascia are elevated medially and laterally off the muscle. Distal tendons are divided and sewn together to avoid shearing the blood supply during harvest. The flap must be elevated off the quadratus plantaris muscle. Finally, the pedicle can be dissected to the origin of the lateral plantar artery in the tarsal tunnel [14].

The reverse-flow flap receives blood supply from the lateral plantar artery via the dorsalis pedis artery and accompanying veins [16]. The skin is incised from the medial malleolus to the midline of the sole, and the abductor hallucis muscle is released from its origin to expose the posterior tibial artery. The bifurcation of the medial and lateral plantar arteries may then be exposed. The lateral plantar artery runs between the flexor digitorum brevis and the quadratus plantae, giving several branches to the flexor digitorum brevis and abductor digiti minimi muscles. Following the pedicle, the flexor digitorum brevis muscle is exposed and disoriginated, leaving the plantar aponeurosis intact. The lateral plantar artery then divides to a superficial and deep branch. The deep branch forms a plantar arch and anastomosis with the deep plantar branch of the dorsalis pedis artery [16]. The distal insertions of the muscle may then be divided and sutured to protect the vascular supply from shearing. Care should be taken to dissect the deep anastomosis away from surrounding tissue to facilitate rotation without kinking.

Wound Closure

The donor site may be closed primarily over a small drain, with plans to remove it the next day. If the donor site has a defect, then a split-thickness skin graft will be needed for coverage of the defect. Flaps should be protected by immobilization with a splint. The limb should be non-weight-bearing and elevated to limit postoperative swelling, which can lead to flap failure. Alternatively, an Ilizarov frame can be employed to offload the flap until it heals in 3–4 weeks.

References

1. Krag C, Riegels-Nielsen P. The dorsalis pedis flap for lower leg reconstruction. Acta Orthop Scand. 1982;53:487–93. https://doi.org/10.3109/17453678208992246.
2. Chandra V, Singh RK. Dorsalis pedis artery-based flap to cover nonhealing wounds over the tendo achillis—a case series. J Orthop Trauma Rehabil. 2017;22:18–21. https://doi.org/10.1016/j.jotr.2015.12.004.

3. McCraw JB, Furlow LT. The dorsalis pedis arterialized flap. A clinical study. Plast Reconstr Surg. 1975;55:177–85.
4. Emsen IM. Reconstruction with distally based dorsalis pedis fasciocutaneous flap for the coverage of distal toe-plantar defects. Can J Plast Surg. 2012;20:e25–7.
5. Özkaya Ö, Yasak T, Üsçetin İ, Kayadibi T. Reversed first dorsal metatarsal artery island flap for first ray defects. J Foot Ankle Surg. 2018;57:184–7. https://doi.org/10.1053/j.jfas.2017.07.013.
6. Beidas OE, Tan BK, Petersen JD. The rotational advancement of medial plantar flap for coverage of foot defect: a case report. Microsurgery. 2012;32:322–5. https://doi.org/10.1002/micr.21956.
7. Schwarz R, Negrini J-F. Medial plantar artery island flap for heel reconstruction. Ann Plast Surg. 2006;57:658–61. https://doi.org/10.1097/01.sap.0000235426.53175.e3.
8. Siddiqi MA, Hafeez K, Cheema TA, Rashid H. The medial plantar artery flap: a series of cases over 14 years. J Foot Ankle Surg. 2012;51:790–4. https://doi.org/10.1053/j.jfas.2012.06.003.
9. Mourougayan V. Medial plantar artery (instep flap) flap. Ann Plast Surg. 2006;56:160. https://doi.org/10.1097/01.sap.0000190830.71132.b8.
10. Harrison DH, Morgan BDG. The instep island flap to resurface plantar defects. Br J Plast Surg. 1981;34:315–8. https://doi.org/10.1016/0007-1226(81)90019-9.
11. Koshima I, Narushima M, Mihara M, Nakai I, Akazawa S, Fukuda N, et al. Island medial plantar artery perforator flap for reconstruction of plantar defects. Ann Plast Surg. 2007;59:558–62.
12. Attinger C, Ducic I, Cooper P, Zelen C. The role of intrinsic muscle flaps of the foot for bone coverage in foot and ankle defects in diabetic and nondiabetic patients. Plast Reconstr Surg. 2002;110:1047–54.
13. Hartrampf CRJ, Scheflan M, Bostwick JI. The flexor digitorum brevis muscle island pedicle flap: a new dimension in heel reconstruction. Plast Reconstr Surg. 1980;66:264.
14. Wei FC, Mardini S. Flaps and reconstructive surgery. 2nd ed. Philadelphia: Elsevier; 2017.
15. Ikuta Y, Murakami T, Yoshioka K, Tsuge K. Reconstruction of the heel pad by flexor digitorum brevis musculocutaneous flap transfer. Plast Reconstr Surg. 1984;74:86–94.
16. Sakai N, Yoshida T, Okumura H. Distal plantar area reconstruction using a flexor digitorum brevis muscle flap with reverse-flow lateral plantar artery. Br J Plast Surg. 2001;54:170–3. https://doi.org/10.1054/bjps.2000.3496.

Chapter 24
Recipient Vessels for Lower Extremity Free Flap Reconstruction

Kate B. Krucoff and Scott T. Hollenbeck

Wounds in the lower extremity may not be amenable to coverage with local tissue. In these instances, free tissue transfer is needed. Finding suitable recipient blood vessels for a microsurgical anastomosis is critical to success. Arterial inflow may be limited because of trauma or atherosclerotic disease. An angiogram can serve as a vascular roadmap for assessing recipient vessels. In general, when large vessels are used as recipient sites, a side branch of the main vessel can be used in an end-to-end fashion. If there are no available side branches, an end-to-side or end-to-end anastomosis to the main vessels may be performed. A thorough vascular exam must be done prior to sacrificing a large artery in the leg. In the lower leg, the tibial vessels are often used in an end-to-end or end-to-side fashion, depending on the overall vascular status.

K. B. Krucoff · S. T. Hollenbeck (✉)
Division of Plastic and Reconstructive Surgery, Duke University Medical Center, Durham, NC, USA
e-mail: scott.hollenbeck@duke.edu

S. T. Hollenbeck et al. (eds.), *Handbook of Lower Extremity Reconstruction*, https://doi.org/10.1007/978-3-030-41035-3_24

At times, an injured artery may be used for inflow. In this instance, the injured vessel is identified and dissected proximally out of the zone of injury until a fully patent vessel is identified. This allows for end-to-end anastomosis without concern for additional loss of distal flow. Likewise, deep venous thrombosis can cause challenges in establishing flap outflow. If this is encountered throughout the leg, free tissue transfer is not possible. Ideally, this condition would be identified preoperatively so that anticoagulation could precede any free flap attempts. In the setting of trauma, superficial veins are often thrombosed, further complicating outflow options. Most major leg arteries are accompanied by two venae comitantes, which are ideal for the venous anastomoses.

Overview of the Medial Thigh

Complex defects of the medial thigh may at times require free tissue transfer. There are numerous recipient vessel options, including the common femoral and superficial femoral vessels. Smaller branches for microsurgical anastomosis include the deep inferior epigastric system and the medial circumflex femoral vessels.

Overview of the Lateral Thigh and Lateral Circumflex Femoral Vessels

Complex defects of the lateral thigh and hip may infrequently require free tissue transfer. The lateral circumflex femoral system is ideal as a recipient site for flap transfer (Fig. 24.1). Also, the descending branch of the lateral circumflex femoral system may be used as an arterial/venous graft.

Overview of the Distal Thigh and Knee

Complex defects involving the knee are somewhat rare, but they are often associated with bony defects, so free tissue

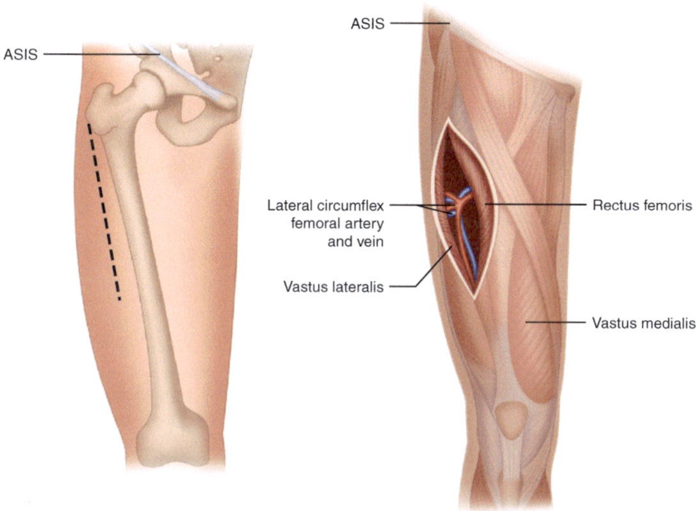

FIGURE 24.1 Preparation of the lateral circumflex femoral vessels. The lateral circumflex femoral vessel system is ideal for microsurgical anastomosis. There are multiple branches that may be used as the primary inflow and outflow. (**a**) An incision is made along a line between the anterior superior iliac spine (ASIS) and the superior lateral aspect of the patella. This is the typical location of the interval between the rectus femoris and the vastus lateralis. (**b**) Once the rectus femoris and vastus lateralis muscles have been separated, the descending branch of the lateral circumflex femoral vessels is seen. The exposure can proceed more proximally to allow for increased vessel size

transfer may be required when local options are not available. There are several options for microsurgical recipient vessels in and around the knee, including the descending branch of the lateral circumflex femoral vessels, the superficial femoral artery, the descending genicular vessels, the popliteal vessels and associated branches, and the anterior or posterior tibial vessels in the lower leg (Fig. 24.2). The decision about which set of vessels to use is usually dependent on patient positioning and concomitant injuries, which may have compromised remote areas.

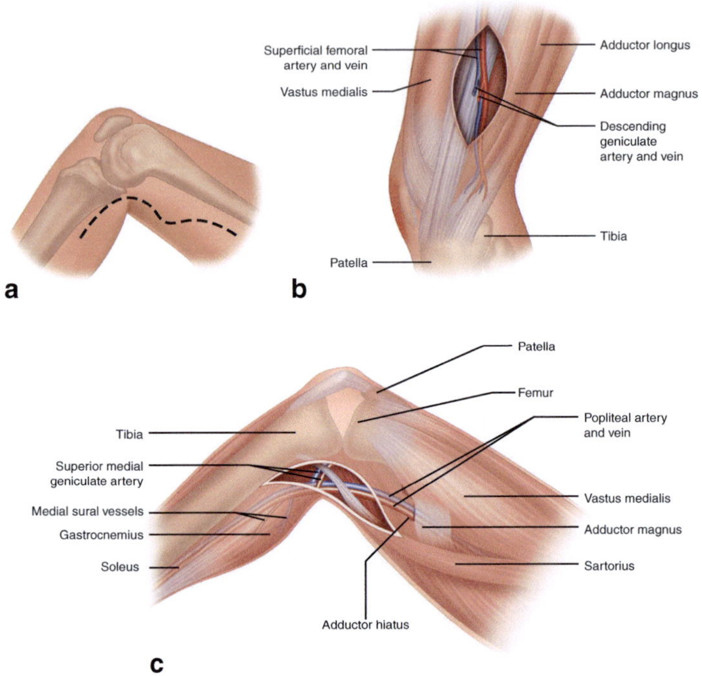

FIGURE 24.2 Preparation of vessels around the knee. (**a**) For this right leg, the hip is externally rotated so that the medial knee is seen. An incision line that starts on the anterior-medial thigh and runs towards the medial-posterior knee is useful for access to superficial femoral vessels and the popliteal vessels. (**b**) A skin incision has been made in the distal aspect of the medial thigh. The dissection has continued down to the interval between the adductor muscles and the vastus medialis. The sartorius muscle has been reflected from medial to lateral. The superficial femoral vessels are seen, in addition to the takeoff of the descending geniculate vessels. Just distal to the takeoff of the geniculate vessels, the superficial femoral artery will dive into the adductor hiatus. (**c**) The posterior-medial thigh skin has been opened to allow for visualization of the popliteal vessels as they exit the adductor hiatus. The superior medial geniculate vessels are seen branching from the popliteal vessels. Distal to this, the medial sural vessels are seen branching from the popliteal vessels. If branches are not available, an end-to-side anastomosis to the popliteal vessels can be performed. The tendons of the sartorius muscle and the hamstring muscles can be seen attaching to the tibia

Overview of the Anterior Lower Leg

Complex wounds of the lower leg are frequently anterior, given the proximity of the tibia bone to the skin. High-energy wounds often require free tissue transfer because of a lack of local flap options. The anterior tibial and posterior tibial vessels are common recipient vessels for free tissue transfer (Fig. 24.3). When dissecting out the anterior tibial vessels, extension of the knee and internal rotation of the leg may be helpful. The dorsalis pedis artery, which is the distal continuation of the anterior tibial artery, also may be used as a recipient vessel. The dorsalis pedis artery can be easily palpated on the proximal aspect of the dorsal foot prior to tourniquet inflation. In some circumstances, the recipient vessels may be distal to the zone of injury. This approach should be used with caution, as intact venous outflow may be limited.

Overview of the Medial Lower Leg

The posterior tibial vessels are the major recipient vessels in the medial leg. The leg can be externally rotated to aid in dissection of the vessels. Additionally, a surgical bump may be placed under the thigh to allow the muscles of the posterior compartment to fall away from the tibia and the underlying posterior tibial vessels. The easiest location for identification of the vessels is just posterior to the medial malleolus at the ankle in the superficial subcutaneous plane (Fig. 24.4). As the vessels are dissected more proximally, their course becomes deeper.

During dissection, care should be taken to avoid injury to the small and great saphenous veins in order to preserve back-up flap venous outflow options. Additionally, the saphenous veins may need to be harvested as vein grafts if surgical dissection finds that the zone of injury to the posterior tibial vessels is extensive.

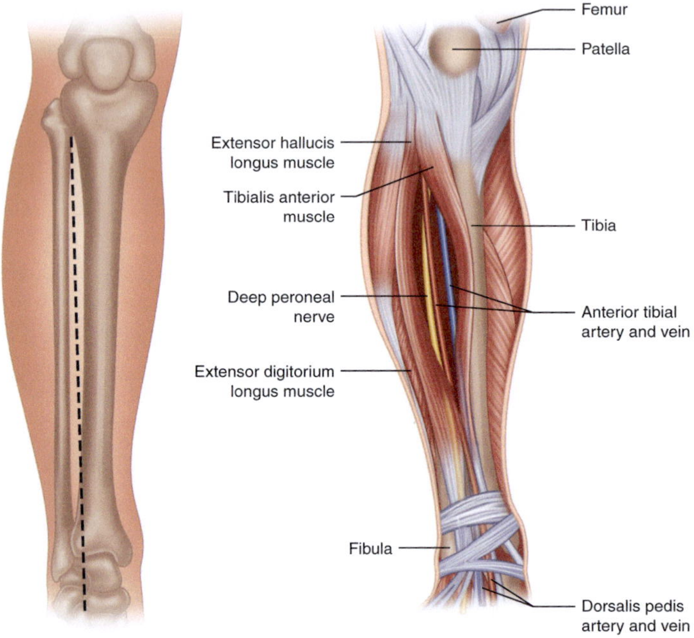

Figure 24.3 Preparation of the anterior tibial and dorsalis pedis vessels. (**a**) An incision that starts just lateral to the edge of the tibia and crosses the midline of the leg as it runs distally toward the central portion of the dorsal foot is useful for access to the anterior tibial and dorsalis pedis vessels. (**b**) The anterior tibial vessels course between the extensor hallucis longus muscle laterally and the tibialis anterior muscle medially after passing anteriorly through the interosseous membrane between the tibia and fibula. The deep peroneal nerve courses with the vessels. Distally, the anterior tibial vessels can be seen branching into the dorsalis pedis artery and veins at the ankle just distal to the extensor retinaculum. The dorsalis pedis vessels are positioned between the extensor tendons in the foot

Distal to the ankle, after passing under the flexor retinaculum, the posterior tibial artery branches into the medial and lateral planar vessels that supply the plantar foot. These vessels also may be used as recipient vessels for free tissue transfer in the treatment of distal ankle and foot wounds.

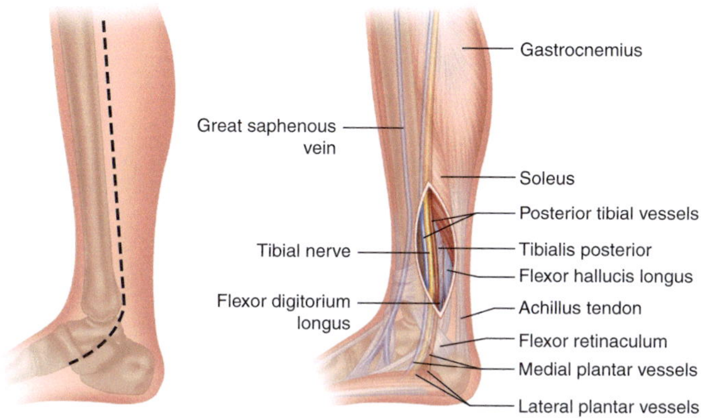

FIGURE 24.4 Preparation of the posterior tibial and plantar vessels. The image shows the medial aspect of a right lower leg. (**a**) An incision line that starts 1–2 cm posterior to the tibia in the proximal leg and runs between the medial malleolus and the Achilles tendon in the distal leg is used to gain access to the posterior tibial vessels. (**b**) A skin incision has been made along the distal lower leg to first identify the posterior tibial vessels and tibial nerve at the ankle, where the neurovascular structures are found superficially, just under the skin. If more proximal access to the vessels is needed, the dissection must proceed deep to the flexor digitorum longus, gastrocnemius, and soleus muscles. The posterior tibial vessels and nerve can then be found coursing along the posterior surface of the deep posterior leg muscles. In the distal ankle, the posterior tibial vessels and nerve can be seen passing through the tarsal tunnel before branching into the medial and lateral plantar arteries and nerves to supply the plantar foot. The roof of the tarsal tunnel, or the flexor retinaculum, can be seen attaching to the distal tibia

Suggested Reading

Fang T, Zhang EW, Lineaweaver WC, Zhang F. Recipient vessels in the free flap reconstruction around the knee. Ann Plastic Surg. 2013;71(4):429–33.

Lorenzo AR, Lin CH, Lin CH, Lin YT, Nguyen A, Hsu C, et al. Selection of the recipient vein in microvascular flap reconstruction of the lower extremity: analysis of 362 free-tissue transfers. J Plast Reconstr Aesthet Surg. 2011;64(5):649–55.

Park S, Han SH, Lee T. Algorithm for recipient vessel selection in free tissue transfer to the lower extremity. Plast Reconstr Surg. 1999;103(7):1937–48.

Index

A
Abductor digiti minimi (ADM) flap, 187
Abductor hallucis (AH) flap, 187
Above-knee amputation (AKA), 197, 205–207
Absolute stability, 56, 59
Adductor/medial compartment of the thigh, 134
Allograft bone, 62
Amputation principles
  energy requirements, 197
  level of, 196–198
  multidisciplinary care, 200
  partial foot amputations, 209
  soft tissue management, 198–200
Angiosome, 116
Ankle
  lower extremity, 36, 37
  skeletal structure, 36
  vascular system, 38, 40
Ankle brachial indexes (ABI), 44
Anterior compartment of the thigh, 133
Anterior cruciate ligament (ACL), 150
Anterior superior iliac spine (ASIS), 227, 253, 297
Anterior tibial artery (ATA), 150, 168
Anterolateral thigh (ALT) flap, 10, 145, 152, 153, 176, 229, 231, 237, 239–243
Autologous bone, 60

B
Below-knee amputation (BKA), 197, 205, 207–209
Bioengineered bi-layered skin, 97
Bioengineered skin, 95
Bipedicled fasciocutaneous flaps, 278
Bipedicled flap, 170, 171, 279
Bone loss, lower extremity injuries
  large-scale defects, 62–64
  small-scale defects, 60–62
Bony reconstruction, 70, 71

C
Celsus, 6
Comminuted fractures, 56
Compartment pressure, 46, 47
Composite vascularized autograft for reconstruction, 72
Critical defects, 60
Cutaneous innervation, 24

S. T. Hollenbeck et al. (eds.), *Handbook of Lower Extremity Reconstruction*, https://doi.org/10.1007/978-3-030-41035-3

Cutaneous reconstruction of the lower extremity, 75

D

Dead space reconstruction, 75
Deep peroneal nerve, 35
Dermal scaffolds, 95
Descending branch of the lateral circumflex femoral (DBLCF) vessels, 121
Diabetic limb reconstruction, 79, 80
  diabetic foot, singularity of, 80, 81
  diabetic vasculopathy, 81, 82
  flap coverage timing, 84
  infection and inflammation, 82
    antibiotics, use of, 83, 84
    serial surgical débridement with tissue culture, 82, 83
  patient selection, 90
  soft tissue reconstruction, 85
    flap selection, 88
    microanastomosis and vessel insetting, 88, 90
    recipient vessel selection, 86, 88
Diabetic vasculopathy, 81, 82
Distal thigh and proximal knee
  lateral thigh propeller flap, 249
  medial thigh propeller flap, 249, 251
  reverse ALT flap, 253–255
  saphenous flap, 246–248
Distal third of lower extremity
  anatomy of, 168, 169
  bipedicled flap, 170, 171
  cross-sectional anatomy, 168
  free ALT flap, 177
  free flaps *vs.* local flaps, 170
  free tissue transfer, 175–177
  keystone flap, 174
  local and regional flaps, 170, 172
  postoperative care, 179
  PPFs, 174
  propeller flap, 174
  reverse sural flap, 172, 173
Distal third tibia
  bipedicled fasciocutaneous flaps, 278, 279
  distal third tibia wound, 274
  keystone flap, 281, 282
  local transposition and rotational flaps, 278
  propeller flap, 279–281
  reverse sural flap, 275–277
Distal third tibia wound, 274
Distraction osteogenesis, 63
Dorsalis pedis flap, 286–289

E

Extensor hallucis longus (EHL), 168
External fixation, 57, 59

F

Fasciocutaneous/adipofascial flap, 102, 104, 161, 162, 176
Fasciocutaneous lower extremity free flaps, 103
Fasciocutaneous perforator flaps, 176
Femoral nerve, 23
Flexor digitorum brevis (FDB) flap, 187, 291–293
Flexor digitorum longus, 137
Flexor retinaculum, 36
Foot
  anatomy and function, 182
  dorsal foot, flaps for, 189–190
  dorsalis pedis flap, 286–289
  flexor digitorum brevis flap, 291–293

free flap
heel, 188
vs. local flaps, 182, 183
options, 185
heel
local and regional flaps, 185, 187
perforator flap, 188
traumatic defect, 191
lower extremity, 36, 37
medial plantar flap, 190, 289–291
muscles of sole, 38–40
musculature, 37, 38
postoperative care, 190–191
skeletal structure, 36
vascular system, 38, 40
Fracture fixation, 56–58
Free anterolateral thigh (ALT) flap, 177
Free flap coverage, 9

G
Gastrocnemius flap, 260
Gastrocnemius muscle, 137
Godina method, 8
Gracilis flap, 220–227
Gracilis muscle, 21, 134
Greater saphenous vein, 41
Gustilo-Anderson classification, 159
Gustilo classification system, 159

H
Hamstrings, 20
Hypercoagulable disorders, 105

I
Immobilization, 56
Induced-membrane technique, 62, 63
Infected Achilles tendon, 94
Investing fascia of the thigh/fascia lata, 14
Ipsilateral free osteocutaneous fibula flap, 109

K
Keystone flap, 174, 281, 282
Knee and proximal lower leg wounds
anatomy and function, 149, 150
complications, 154
extensor mechanism injuries, 154
free tissue transfer, 154
muscle and fasciocutaneous flaps, 150–153
postoperative care, 154
Knee and proximal tibia, soft tissue reconstruction, 258–261

L
Lateral circumflex arterial system, 22
Lateral circumflex femoral artery (LCFA), 231, 240
Lateral collateral ligament (LCL), 150
Lateral gastrocnemius flap, 152
Lateral thigh and hip
ALT flap, 239–243
TFL flap, 239
Leg
fascial layers, 25
innervation, 34, 35
musculature, 25, 30–32
skeletal structure, 24
vascular system, 32, 33
Leg muscles, 29, 30
Leg musculature, 25–28, 30–32
Lessor saphenous vein, 41
Limb-threatening ischemia, 47

Local muscle flaps, 187
lower leg, 134, 136, 137
Mathes and Nahai muscle classification, 131, 132
pedicled muscle flap, 133
principles of, 129, 130
upper leg, 133, 134
Lower extremity
acute trauma, external fixation, 59
ankle and foot
fascial layers, 36, 37
foot musculature, 37, 38
innervation, 41
leg musculature, 26–28
skeletal structure, 36
thigh musculature, 16–18
vascular system, 38, 40
venous anatomy, 41
bone loss after trauma, 60
large-scale defects, 62–64
small-scale defects, 60–62
fracture fixation, 55–58
free flap reconstruction
anterior lower leg, 299
anterior tibial and dorsalis pedis vessels, 300
distal thigh and knee, 296–299
lateral circumflex femoral vessels, 297
lateral thigh and lateral circumflex femoral vessels, 296
medial lower leg, 299–300
medial thigh, 296
posterior tibial and plantar vessels, 301
leg, 24
fascial layers, 25
innervation, 34, 35
musculature, 25, 30–32
skeletal structure, 24
vascular system, 32, 33
local skin flaps, 117
delay principles, 117, 118
geometric design of flaps, 121
perforator flaps, 118
perfusion of skin, 116
principles, 116
reverse flaps, 120
osseous healing, 58, 59
reconstruction, 4, 101
advances in field, 8, 9, 11
bioengineered skin, 95
dermal scaffolds, 95
flap timing, 104
free flap approach, 108, 110
free flaps, technical considerations for, 110, 111
historical perspectives, 4, 6, 8
intraoperative thrombotic complications, 107
local *vs.* free flaps, 105
muscle *vs.* fasciocutaneous flaps, 102, 104
NPWT devices, 94
placenta-derived constructs, 95
postoperative care, 111–113
tape dermatogenesis and tissue expansion, 95
thigh, 13
fascial layers, 14
innervation, 23, 24
musculature, 15, 21
skeletal structure, 14
vascular system, 21–23
Lower leg, 134, 136, 137

M
Massive osteocutaneous defects, 70
Mathes and Nahai flap, 152, 161

muscle flap, 150
type II flap, 264
type IV flap, 268
Medial and lateral thigh propeller flap, 249
Medial circumflex femoral artery, 22
Medial collateral ligament (MCL), 149–150
Medial gastrocnemius flap, 151
Medial plantar flap, 289–291
Medial sural artery perforator (mSAP) flap, 151, 258–261
Medial thigh and groin
ALT flap, 229, 231, 232, 234, 235
gracilis flap, 220–227
rectus femoris flap, 227, 229, 230, 232
sartorius flap, 217–221
Medial thigh propeller flap, 251
Microanastomosis, 88, 90
Middle third of leg
anatomy and function, 158, 159
Gustilo-Anderson cassification, 159
muscle and fasciocutaneous flaps, 161
omentum free flap, 163
perforator flaps for, 162, 163
soleus flap, 160
Middle third of tibia
soleus flap, 264–268
tibialis anterior flap, 268–270
Muscle flaps, 102, 104, 161, 176
Muscular reconstruction, 73, 74

N
Negative pressure wound therapy (NPWT), 9, 51, 94, 104, 206
Neovascularization, 117
Nerve reconstruction, 74, 75

O
Obturator nerve, 24
Omentum free flap, 163
Oncologic defect reconstruction, 67–70
arterial and venous reconstruction, 74
bony reconstruction, 70, 71
cutaneous reconstruction, 75, 76
dead space reconstruction and prosthesis coverage, 75, 76
muscular reconstruction, 73, 74
nerve reconstruction, 74, 75
postoperative care, 76
soft tissue reconstruction, 71, 73
Open fractures, 159
Orthopedic fixation, 47
Orthoplastic surgery, 6, 9
Osseous healing, 58, 59
Osteoconduction, 60
Osteogenesis, 60
Osteoinduction, 60
Osteomyelitis, 49

P
Parascapular flaps, 178
Partial foot amputations, 209
Pedicled gastrocnemius flap, 137
Pedicled muscle flap, 133
Pedicled perforator flaps (PPFs), 174
Perforator flaps, 118
Peroneal nerve curves, 34
Peroneal retinaculum, 36
Placenta-derived constructs, 95
Plantar fascia, 36
Posterior compartment, 134

Posterior cruciate ligament (PCL), 150
Posterior femoral cutaneous nerves (PFCN), 35, 206
Posterior tibial (PT) artery, 137, 169, 267
Postoperative care, 76, 111
Profunda femoris, 22
Propeller flap, 120, 174, 279–281
Punctate bone bleeding, 47

Q
Quadriceps muscle, 15

R
Radial forearm free flap, 192
Radiation, 73
Reconstructive microsurgery, 8
Rectus femoris flap, 134, 144, 227, 229
Relative stability, 58
Reverse anterolateral thigh (ALT) flap, 253–255
Reverse flaps, 120
Reverse sural flap, 119, 172, 173, 186, 275–277

S
Saphenous flap, 246–248
Saphenous nerve, 35
Sarcoid ulcer, 99
Sartorius flap, 143, 217
Sartorius muscle, 15
Sciatic nerve, 23, 34, 35
Soft tissue reconstruction
    diabetic limb reconstruction, 79, 80, 85
        flap selection, 88
        microanastomosis and vessel insetting, 88, 90
        recipient vessel selection, 86, 88
    distal thigh and proximal knee
        medial and lateral thigh propeller flap, 249
        medial thigh propeller flap, 251
        reverse ALT flap, 253–255
        saphenous flap, 246–248
    distal third of lower extremity
        anatomy of, 168, 169
        bipedicled flap, 170, 171
        cross-sectional anatomy, 168
        free ALT flap, 177
        free flaps *vs*. local flaps, 170
        free tissue transfer, 175–177
        keystone flap, 174
        local and regional flaps, 170, 172
        postoperative care, 179
        PPFs, 174
        propeller flap, 174
        reverse sural flap, 172, 173
    distal third tibia
        bipedicled fasciocutaneous flaps, 278
        bipedicled flap, 279
        distal third tibia wound, 274
        keystone flap, 281, 282
        local transposition and rotational flaps, 278
        propeller flap, 279–281
        reverse sural flap, 275–277
    foot
        anatomy and function, 182
        dorsal foot, flaps for, 189–190
        dorsalis pedis flap, 286–289
        flexor digitorum brevis flap, 291–293
        free flaps *vs*. local flaps, 182, 183

free flap options, 185
heel, free flaps for, 188
heel, local and regional flaps, 185, 187
heel, perforator flap, 188
heel, traumatic defect, 191
medial plantar flap, 190, 289–291
postoperative care, 190–191
lateral thigh and hip
ALT flap, 239–243
TFL flap, 239
middle third of tibia
soleus flap, 264–268
tibialis anterior flap, 268–270
mSAP flap, knee and proximal tibia, 258–261
medial thigh and groin
ALT flap, 229, 231, 232, 234, 235
gracilis flap, 220–227
rectus femoris flap, 227, 229, 230, 232
sartorius flap, 217–221
middle third of leg
anatomy and function, 158, 159
Gustilo-Anderson cassification, 159
muscle and fasciocutaneous flaps, 161
omentum free flap, 163
perforator flaps for, 162, 163
soleus flap, 160
middle third of tibia
soleus flap, 264–268
tibialis anterior flap, 268–270
Soft tissue sarcomas, 71
Soleus flap, 160, 264, 265, 267, 268
Soleus muscle, 137
Superficial fascia, 14
Superficial femoral artery, 22, 150
Superficial peroneal nerve, 35
Superficial toe ulcer, 97, 98
Superior lateral genicular artery, 32
Supermicrosurgery, 87
Sural nerve, 35

T

Tape dermatogenesis, 95
Targeted muscle reinnervation (TMR), 199–203, 208
Tensor fascia lata (TFL) flap, 237, 239
Thigh innervation, 23, 24
Thigh musculature, 15–18, 21
Thigh soft tissue reconstruction, 13
ALT flap, 145
anatomy and function, 140, 141
fascial layers, 14
innervation, 23, 24
local flaps
free flaps *vs.*, 141
for groin reconstruction, 142, 144, 145
for Hip, 141, 142
for upper knee, 146
muscles of, 19
musculature, 15, 21
rectus femoris flap, 144
sartorius flap, 143
skeletal structure, 14
vascular system, 21–23
Thigh vascular system, 21–23
3 reverse sural flap, 172
Through-knee amputation (TKA), 197
Tibial artery, 32
Tibialis anterior (TA), 269
Tissue allotransplantation, 11
Tissue expansion, lower extremity reconstruction, 95

Transosseus myodesis, 199
Transpelvic amputations, 204, 205
Transposition flap, 123
Traumatic hip disarticulations, 204, 205
Traumatized leg
- acute trauma principles, 44
- compartment pressure evaluation and treatment, 46, 47
- osteomyelitis, 49
- reconstruction timing, 51–53
- vascular and orthopedic intervention, 47

U

Upper leg, 133

V

V.A.C. VERAFLO™ device, 94
Vascularized autograft, 63
Vastus lateralis, 134
Venous thromboembolism (VTE), 52

MIX
Papier aus verantwortungsvollen Quellen
Paper from responsible sources
FSC® C105338

If you have any concerns about our products,
you can contact us on
ProductSafety@springernature.com

In case Publisher is established outside the EU,
the EU authorized representative is:
Springer Nature Customer Service Center GmbH
Europaplatz 3, 69115 Heidelberg, Germany

Printed by Libri Plureos GmbH
in Hamburg, Germany